How To Bottom Like a Porn Star

by Woody Miller

WOODPECKER**MEDIA**

Print layout by eBooks by Barb
for booknook.biz

INTRODUCTION

Have you ever looked at gay porn and thought, "How can they make bottoming look so easy?" A hung top sticks it in like a glute inject and the bottom doesn't even flinch. How do porn star bottoms do it? And more importantly, what can you learn from them so that you can, too?

There are a lot of lessons to be learned from gay porn, both good and bad. This book exposes the shockingly stupid, medically dangerous tactics that porn stars use to bottom without pain, highlights many of the things they do correctly and outlines a step-by-step plan that will help you enjoy a lifetime of painless bottoming.

Before we get started, let me explain how I got the information you're about to read. I commissioned a team of researchers to interview a truckload of gay porn industry folk—cameramen, scouts, producers, directors and performers. Most turned us down, for fear of retribution that might come from airing the porn industry's secrets. We had to promise complete anonymity and therefore you will not see any recognizable names, though we interviewed many of the giants of the industry.

Many of the porn star secrets to bottoming without pain are so shockingly dangerous they posed an ethical dilemma for me: Do I tell you what they are knowing that no matter how I frame my warnings, a certain percentage of you will go ahead and try their risky tactics?

In the end I decided that honesty was the best way to approach my dilemma. Yes, some readers won't care about the risks, just as some people try smoking after they read the warning label. I thought of titling this book, *How To Bottom Like A Porn Star Without Resorting To Dangerous Methods*, but my editor told me to quit whimpering and take it like a man. Guess we know who the top is in that relationship! The truth is, porn star bottoms have a lot to teach us, and as long as you know what is acceptable from a common-sense standpoint, the truth shall be told.

So, let's have some fun! You're about to get some fascinating, behind-the-scenes, no-holds-barred insights into an industry that we've all helped make rich, and on the way you are going to learn how to bottom without pain so you can screw like a porn star.

Let's start at the beginning.

Millions of gay men can't seem to get past their physical and psychological stumbling blocks to enjoy the intense ecstasy that bottoming can provide. This is a shame because as you've seen in gay porn, you can *easily* bottom without pain. In fact, I used the sensible aspects of porn star bottoming and combined them with recommendations from a team of experts, including a yoga guru, a respiratory psychophysiologist, a colo-rectal specialist and a physician with a masterful knowledge of anatomy to create an easy-to-follow guide to bottoming without pain.

Bottoming isn't just about the physical sensation of being penetrated. It's the emotional high of accepting someone else's presence in your body. It's the psychological thrill of being momentarily "owned," of submitting yourself to the strength of another man. If you're in a relationship it's the ultimate act of union. If you're single it's a hot way of having fun. And if you're a newbie, it's an act that fear and pain prevent you from completing. If you bought this book you probably fall into one of two types of guys:

1. **You Really Want To Bottom But You're Too Afraid To Try.** You just can't imagine how something so big can fit into such a little hole without causing an excruciating amount of pain. You're probably also afraid of the mess you might leave behind on the sheets. Some guys live in mortal fear that bottoming will create a "shit show" in the bedroom and stain their psyches as well as their sheets.

2. **You've Tried Bottoming And It Hurt Like Hell.** In fact, it was as painful as you feared and while there wasn't a shit show, there was the odd smell or tire track that kinda grossed you out. You stopped trying even though still, to this day, you want to have the experience of pain-free, pleasure-filled bottoming.

Pain, or the fear of pain, is the biggest reason gay men shy away from bottoming. It doesn't have to be that way. The only reason it hurts so much is that you don't understand the three sources of pain and how to avoid them. In this book I'm going to show you specific techniques that will allow you to experience the ecstasy of bottoming without any of the pain you've come to fear or associate with it.

Bottoming is not the sexual equivalent of walking over hot coals. You don't have to put yourself through hell to get to the other side. You just have to follow the plan I've developed with the help of respected medical experts in the field of urology, proctology, yoga, psychology and gastroenterology.

I've been writing about gay sex for over ten years. I starred in an international hit TV show called *The Sex Inspectors* (it aired in 12 countries, including the U.S. (HBO) and the U.K. (Channel Four). I've also written several sex books and write a popular, syn-dicated gay sex column called *Need Wood? Tips For Getting Timber.*

I've answered thousands of questions over the course of my career and if there's one thing I've learned it's that gay men don't want acres and acres of explanation before getting down to essential information. That's why you'll notice that this is a short book. This is not an accident. I know when you ask for the time you don't want to know how the watch was built. And so I've limited the information in this book strictly to answering a single question: How can you bottom like a porn star without pain or stains? If you want the history of enemas, a guide to anal wellness, an explan-ation of sexually transmitted diseases or the general care and feeding of the gluteus maximus you're out of luck.

Before we get started, let's take a look at how this book is laid out, chapter by chapter:

TABLE OF CONTENTS

CHAPTER ONE

The Porn Star Bottom.
A Spread-Eagled View.

IN THE PORN INDUSTRY, the hard work for the "receiver" is in the lead-up rather than during the actual shoot. The most obvious priority is getting your anal area prepped so that no unexpected co-stars make a cameo appearance. Whether bottoming on camera or in the privacy of your bedroom, one should always be conscious of his diet, but this is particularly important in the days leading up to a porn shoot.

In the two or three days before the filming, many porn bottoms stick to a high-fiber, low carb diet. It's lots of fruits and vegetables, with plenty of juices and water (you're getting ready to spend several hours under blazing hot spotlights, so it's important to be hydrated). Chicken and fish are preferred proteins because white meat is lighter than red meat, although some bottoms swear off all pork to decrease the likelihood of "bacon bits."

A proper diet gets your butt halfway to Hollywood, but to make sure your butt is ready to catch big cargo on cam it's also good to warm it up beforehand. Prior to a shoot, usually the evening before or morning of, it's not uncommon for porn bottoms to calibrate their sphincters by inserting a dildo or small butt plug for a few hours to make sure their starfish is camera-ready.

The morning of the shoot should start with a good bowel movement. Many porn bottoms have their superstitions for what cleans them out thoroughly: for some it's a cigarette, for others it's a large coffee or smoothie.

After the morning dump, it's time to start douching (although some porn bottoms start this process the night before, especially if they're prepping for a gang bang scene). They douche early and douche often. They do not to stop at the first sight of clear liquid coming out of their bum. Bottoming on camera requires DEEP cleaning; so proper douching can be a multi-hour project.

As High As A California Redwood. If porn star A does 3 lines of crystal meth and porn star B does 6 lines of meth, how many more lines of meth does B have to do to.... And how many times does he have to bottom to pay for the difference? You don't have to be a genius at math to know that the porn industry is riddled with drugs. One porn star we interviewed estimated that 75% of performers use some combination of poppers, crystal meth, ecstasy, GHB, molly, Viagra, Levitra, Cialis, and the list goes on. *"Usually, we'll do it in the bathroom right before when we are cleaning up [douching],"* said one porn star. *"It's a 'don't ask don't tell' policy kind of. The studio people look the other way. And it's also sort of bonding."*

Studios will publicly deny that there's drug use among performers, or at the very least, deny that they *provide* the drugs. Yet many performers told us that some studios will keep 'emergency' erectile dysfunction drugs in case performers forget to bring theirs. It must be said that not all porn performers use drugs but all, *all* the industry folks we talked to said drugs are a huge part of the scene.

Lights, Camera – No Action! Once the cameras are rolling, the hard work shifts to the top, which brings us to a surprising aspect of porn: It takes a lot of time, effort and lubrication to get —and keep —a penis erect on camera (porn shoots take so long the Viagra wears off!). Sure, most gay porn videos go from eye glance to anal penetration in less than ninety seconds, but porn stars never show up to a shoot and start banging instantaneously. It takes a lot of work to make it look effortless.

Being a good porn bottom requires empathy and patience, for it's never productive for them to share how irritated they are that the top can't keep his penis erect. No matter how spontaneous and intense your favorite porn scenes appear, it's guaranteed that they involved a lot of Hurry-Up-And-Wait.

Straight Guys In Gay Porn. One of the most shocking aspects of the gay porn industry is the number of straight performers in it. It's hard to quantify just how many joes are playing mo's because the number depends on whom you ask. There is a wide discrepancy in estimates but of the porn industry folks we interviewed, it ranged from as low as 20% to as high as 50%.

Some gay performers don't think they're all that hetero. One told us, *"No, if those guys are there, they're not really straight. They're turned on by the cameras. It's kind of secretive and dangerous. It's like they're getting away with something that they're not supposed to be doing."*

Still, most gay performers believe there are plenty of hetero performers in gay porn. Which brings us to the question of how straight guys get hard for their gay partners. *"They would prepare the same way as any other guy would prepare,"* one gay performer told us. "But as straight guys, they're more focused on the money, how much money are they going to make rather than will this feel good. They usually have their girlfriend perform them [fluffer] or have straight porn available so they can stay erect."

And what about straight guys bottoming? Here's how one gay porn star answered the question: *"They do use Viagra. And often, the girlfriends are there so if they need a helping hand. The ones there are really understanding, "Okay, this is what my boyfriend does, and he feels comfortable enough for me to support him while watching him." But it really depends on the girl, like your partners in life, it just depends on their character."*

Wax It, Baby. Some studios require, as a standard of performance, to wax your anus. This is changing somewhat as natural hair is beginning to find some popularity. Here's how one performer put it, *"If I bottom for a scene, I wax. I would never shoot a scene if I waxed that day, but I would bottom if I had waxed within seven days of the day that I waxed. I would have a groomer wax. The personal groomer is from the spa, the same guy who does my manicures. It's hard to find somebody though at a legal establishment who is willing to do that kind of personal service as far as waxing goes."*

Split Scenes: The tried-and-true formula of porn —a little bit of kissing leading to a lot of sucking leading to hardcore penetration —is made possible through the magic of editing. Rarely is there a natural transition from one activity to another on a porn set, and many times the opening foreplay is shot after everyone has ejaculated.

In truth, after the oral scenes are shot, there's often a break so that the bottom can douche one final time and the top can pop another Viagra. Once the banging starts, there are frequent time-outs during position changes, and every two-minute clip of different positions —riding, doggie, missionary —can take at least an hour to shoot. If you're an avid porn viewer, I'm sure you've caught lapses in continuity, like, "Was he wearing these boots ten seconds ago?"

Lastly, a top rarely pulls out and delivers the money shot without a fair amount of time in unseen masturbating, and making it appear otherwise is how video editors make their money.

A Minute Takes An Hour To Shoot. Porn videos are heavily edited. *Heavily.* Unless the studio is a we-don't-care-how-it-looks-get-it-out-the-door chop shop, it typically takes between five and eight hours to shoot a typical screwing scene. Even a simple blowjob scene takes an average of about two hours to film. One famous director put it this way: *"There's no formula. It really just varies from director to director. But on* *average, I would say that it could probably take 4-6 hours to produce 30 minutes of usable tape."*

Faking It: Bottoms are the only real actors on a porn shoot, and most times their work is worthy of an Academy Award. Let's start with analingus: Yes, there are some world-class kitchen cleaners in the porn industry, but a lot of the tops in porn are too selfish to do it regularly, and so you get a lot of guys who are amateurs. They're only doing tongue duty because the director told them to, or because they're trying to dis - tract attention away from their limp penises.

The same goes for going wild while bottoming: The porn star bottom has to make viewers feel like their insides are throbbing, and leave them unaware that they've taken shits that were more painful and/or pleasurable than the banging they're re - ceiving right now.

In other words, when you see a porn star bottom in pain, *he's acting.* He's not in any kind of pain; it's just an act to fulfill the viewer fantasy of giving or receiving pain and make the viewer feel like the top is bigger than he is in reality.

Sleight Of Hand: If online dating has taught us anything, it's that any penis can look hard and humongous from the right angle. In porn, it can take hours to find that proper angle, and the goal of most shoots is to find a few clusters of useable footage from the hours spent producing a scene. This is when the porn bottom becomes a physical artist, as a cocked leg or hyper-pronounced back arch can be more visually flattering than the footage would look from standard doggie-style.

Other visual tricks involve concealing the bottom's own limp penis, which is usually accomplished simply with hands or a jock strap. Although a standard in real-world gay sex, poppers somehow ruin the primal facade of porn, so it also takes focus to use them discreetly and keep them off camera.

Gang Bang Roulette: The hottest action in a lot of gangbang scenes are often not caught on camera. There's usually a lot of fluffing going on among the tops in a gang bang scene, mainly to get each other hard enough (long enough) to plow the on-screen bottom. Also, the hottest packing the bottom receives can often come from unexpected sources such as another porn star who is primarily known as a power bottom, or even the cameraman or associate producer.

Shits And Giggles. Sometimes tension relief on the set comes in the form of comedy. One time, a performer told us, *"I fell off the table when the guy fucked me so hard and*

I busted my head open. I had to go to the hospital. But watching it was hilarious as hell."

What Do Gay Porn Stars Earn? Remarkably little. While some name brand stars can earn up to $5,000 a scene, the vast majority make about $500 to $1,000 per scene. No matter how you do the math, that doesn't come to a whole lot of money. Very few performers make a living off of porn. Most use it as a way to supplement the income they make from their day jobs or as a way to jack up their prostitution rates. They can charge a lot more money if customers perceive them as porn stars.

Do tops make more money than bottoms? The industry folks we spoke to said top and bottom don't matter nearly as much as celebrity status. The more well-known you are the more money you're going to command, no matter what position you take during filming. Some folks told us tops tend to make more because the penis is always the star of the show and that they've got to stay hard for hours on end. But some said bottoms make more because they're at a much higher risk for HIV and as one performer charmingly put it, *"We have to keep our holes gaping open all day."*

The After-Party: Besides heading to the bank as soon as possible to make sure the check clears from the porn studio, the first priority of many porn bottoms is to soak in a hot bath of Epsom salts. Getting your butt played with and stretched open for hours can cause some serious rectal inflammation, and post-bottoming care is essential to make sure the next time a director yells, "Action!" it doesn't happen in the Emergency Room.

It's A Wrap! Now that you've got a good feel about how your favorite porn videos get made, let's take a closer look at how you can bottom like a porn star without be-coming an ER victim. The most important sexual organ is the one between your ears, not your legs. As you'll see in the next chapter, bottoming doesn't start with spread-ing your thighs but opening your mind.

CHAPTER TWO

Free Your Mind,
Your Butt Will Follow

"Anticipatory pain" and a perceived loss of masculinity can put your butt in a headlock. Here's how to resolve the emotional blocks that stop you from trying or enjoying anal sex.

WHEN WAS THE LAST TIME you heard someone make fun of a top? Never. But bottoms? Wow. How many times have you heard friends say things like, *"Oh, he's just a big bottom."* Or heard jokes like, *"Why did the gay man cross the road? He heard the chicken was a top."*

Can you imagine somebody saying, *"There's nothing but tops in this town?"* Exactly. You can't. The most exalted thing you can say about a gay man, the biggest compliment you can pay him, is to call him a "top." And the worst thing you can say about him, the best way to put him down, is to call him a "bottom." Why? Because a lot of people buy into the idea that…

Bottoming Makes You A Woman.

This is the single biggest emotional stumbling block gay men have about bottoming —being labeled less than a man. For many of us, bottoming isn't an opportunity to enjoy a pleasurable sexual experience but an act that threatens our sense of masculinity and the respect that goes with it. Many gay men believe that if they bottom they will become "a bottom." They fear that bottoming will create a new unwanted identity for them; that they'll become, ahem, the butt of everyone's jokes.

It just may be that you haven't been able to bottom (or been able to enjoy it) because you have so many emotional issues around the act. If you can get away from the falsehood of bottoming as an identity and see it for what it is—an erotic activity—the more relaxed and receptive you will be.

It might be helpful to understand how so many of us came to associate bottoming with effeminacy. The answer can be found in one of the most important gay books you'll ever read—historian Byrne Fone's *Homophobia: A History.* He makes well-documented assertions that sex between men in Ancient Greece was "normal" and idealized, but that there were strict rules regarding its conduct. There were Homo Do's and Homo Don'ts. And the biggest Don't was to enjoy penetration.

Being the penetrator was synonymous with being a man. Anything that subverted the concept of masculinity was punished with social ostracism and ridicule. And nothing mocked masculinity more than getting penetrated.

Greeks and Romans didn't really care whom you had sex with (women, men, boys, slaves) as long as you were the penetrator. The Romans even had a word for it: *Vir.*

It was an exalted term, symbolizing the ideal man: He who penetrates other men but is himself not penetrated.

Today we still live out those vestiges of antiquity. We label men "tops" or "bottoms" in part because we're living out antiquity's fear of the feminine. In heterosexual thinking, the penetrator (man) is more valuable than the penetrated (women). We've adapted that consciousness in our own community, where the penetrator (top) is more valuable than the penetrated (bottom).

Clearly, labels like "top" and "bottom" can be useful shorthand for sexual likes and dislikes. But instead of stating what we prefer— "I like to bottom"— we turned that preference into an identity—"I'm a bottom."

By developing identities out of these labels we cut ourselves off of any unlabeled possibilities. In our world, tops can only date or hook up with bottoms and bottoms can only do the same with tops. That's a whole lot of blindness in a sighted community.

I Call Bullshit.

To say that a top is more masculine than a bottom is bullshit. First, the preference for a sexual position says NOTHING about you as a person. Just like your sexual orientation says nothing about your character, your preference for bottoming says nothing about your masculinity.

Labels Belong On Can, Not A Man. I don't like the words "top", "bottom" or even "versatile" because in the end, they're labels. And while labels can sometimes act as helpful linguistic shorthand, they almost always morph into psychic prisons prevent - ing you from experiencing all that there is to experience. There is no shame in being gay; there is no shame in liking to receive. The only thing shameful is how willing we are to buy into such bogus identities. You will note throughout this book that I do not use the words "top" or "bottom" as identities, but as verbs. I do not think you are a "top" because you prefer to insert. I do not think you are a "bottom" because you like to receive. Unless you can start seeing these words as verbs instead of identities, it will be difficult for you to mentally relax enough to bottom without pain.

No amount of sphincter relaxation exercises, breathing patterns and desensitization techniques can overcome a paralyzing fear of losing your masculinity. Unless you come to terms with your fears, unless you start rejecting the demonstrably false belief that receiving a penis makes you less than a man it will be very difficult for you to bottom pleasurably (if at all).

You can't shut off a long-held belief as if it was a light switch, but you can make a lot of progress by questioning the assumptions you've internalized. Let's start with the biggest one. It goes something like this:

1.   Men give their penises.

2.   Women receive them.

3.   Therefore, if you receive a penis between your legs it makes you a woman.

Now, let's test this assumption. Do you like to give oral sex? I'm going to make the fairly safe assumption that you do. Now, do you feel like a woman during or after oral sex? Do you suddenly give up beer for cosmos? Do you give up playing tennis to take up knitting? Do you give up Levi's for Laura Ashley?

Women receive penises in their mouths, too. Does that make you a woman? Now, think about this. If your sense of masculinity isn't threatened by receiving a penis in your mouth (something women do), why would it be threatened by receiving it between your legs (something women do)? They're both orifices. Remember this and whatever emotional block you have about bottoming will slowly disappear:

Masculinity isn't about what you put into your body.
It's about what you put out in the world.

I have a couple of friends who are serious boxers. They both like to bottom. They also like to punch the crap out of their opponents in the ring. Bottoming did not turn them into something they're not. Nothing about who you are or what you're about changes after receiving a penis in your mouth, and nothing will change after you receive on in your butt.

Now, let's tackle another fear that stops guys from even considering the idea of bottoming. It usually comes in the form of a question.

Will I Become An Insatiable Bottom?

Another common belief associated with the "bottoming makes you a woman" myth is that you might like bottoming so much that you'll never want to do anything else. Funny how nobody worries that they'll become an insatiable top. At any rate, the fear of liking the lower bunk a little too much can make you tense up so much that you can't relax enough to enjoy bottoming.

The idea that you'll get trapped by trying something new in bed is yet another sex-negative belief. If you try steak and love it does that mean you'll never eat chicken again? If you see a drama and love it does that mean you'll never watch a comedy again? We are expanded, not trapped, by what we like. And even if you end up pre-ferring to bottom over any other activity, so what? You may as well tell me you've recently discovered that you prefer writing with your left hand, for what it says about you. Adding new experiences to your life doesn't subtract anything from who you are.

Remember, labels belong on a can, not a man. Beware the associations you subconsciously make about sexual positions. Look at the title of this section again ("Will I Become An Insatiable Bottom?"). Would it have struck as much fear in you if I had written, "Will I Become An Insatiable Top?" No, because there is no stigma to topping. But to many gay men, bottoming has a lingering stigma of effeminacy.

Challenge your assumption that bottoming is an identity; that it makes you effeminate, that it's something real men don't do. If it helps, I'll be more than glad to put you in the ring with my boxing friends.

How "Anticipatory Pain" Can Make Your Butt Tighter Than Two Coats Of Paint.

"Anticipatory pain" is a psychological term for the expectation of pain. It speaks to the emotional and physical consequences of this expectation. For example, if you are convinced that something will be painful, your body will tense up in the expectation of it. The more you believe that bottoming will hurt, the tenser your body will get. Your butt will clench for its safety as hard as it can. This expectation of pain contributes greatly to your inability to relax. If you're convinced that bottoming is going to hurt like hell, how in God's pajamas are you going to be relaxed enough to enjoy it? Imagine telling someone, "This is going to hurt worse than a motor-powered root canal, so just relax." Right. That's helpful. But that's what you're saying to yourself and as long as you keep saying it you're destined for failure.

But wait, you say! You've heard horror stories from your friends and hell, it hurts even when you stick your pinky up there—how could a penis NOT hurt going in? Here's how: Because the entire anus, from the sphincter to the anal canal to the rectum, is made up of incredibly supple, flexible muscle and tissue that, with the right conditioning, can stretch and expand way beyond its current size without causing harm or pain. To get a sense of the flexibility in your puborectal region, know this: During rectal surgery your anus can be safely stretched to the point that the surgeon'-s hand can easily pass through the anal canal.

Let's just hope the surgeon doesn't get an attack of jazz hands during the procedure.

With the right conditioning your anal muscles can relax enough to easily accommodate a penis without any pain whatsoever. You see the evidence of this on your computer's hard drive or your Internet browser—where you store, bookmark and view your favorite porn. If you learn anything from porn (other than you like way too much of it!) it's this: With the right approach, you can painlessly take in guys who are hung like the Florida panhandle.

You're going to learn a special new technique I developed to help you do that, but it won't work if you're saddled with the expectation of pain. Fortunately, there's a very easy way to make your belief in misery go away: Commit yourself to a…

No Pain Contract.

It basically states that you will not engage in any sexual activity that causes pain. You refuse to experience anything that hurts, no matter how little it is or how much your partner encourages you to go on. You commit yourself to a program of systematic desensitization: You'll let fingers, toys and penises only go in as far as it feels comfortable then back off. You know this will comfortably stretch you and that the next time you will be able to go in further. You promise to never, EVER to go past your comfort threshold. Not even a little bit. Your No Pain contract is simple: No Pain, No Way, No How, Not Ever.

Sign here.

Now, doesn't that feel like a weight has been lifted off your shoulders? You are not going to experience pain when you bottom. Ever. You have now replaced the expectation of pain with the expectation of NO PAIN. You have now replaced a failed formula (no pain=no gain) with a successful one (no pain=gain). Again, we can look to porn for a great reminder of this. Porn star bottoms are *never* in pain, even when they have huge guys inside them. Several porn directors told us a bottoming scene can take up to eight hours to shoot. There is no way they will allow an inexperienced bottom who hasn't mastered pain-free bottoming on the set. Remember what I said earlier: Bottoming is not the same as walking on hot coals. You don't have to suffer to get to the other side.

Let's Review.

There are two emotional roadblocks that can make bottoming exceedingly difficult: The fear that bottoming will destroy your self-conception and/or that it will be an ex-cruciatingly painful experience. The solutions are simple:

1. **Question the assumptions you've made about receiving a penis.** Giving and receiving are different sides of the male coin. You are not any more male if you top than if you bottom. Bottoming will not strip you of your masculinity.

2. **Mentally sign a No Pain contract.** Your mantra should be no way, no how, not ever. By replacing an expectation of pain with the anticipation of pleasure you will relieve yourself of a tremendous, paralyzing burden that keeps you from bottoming successfully.

Now that we've handled the psychological blocks that might stop you from bottoming, let's talk about the very real physical challenge before you: How do you get something as large as a penis through something as small as your sphincter without excruciating pain?

Easily. By combining the best of porn star approaches with systematic desensitization, progressive muscle relaxation and sexual imagery I've come up with an approach I call the Sexhalation Method. Before I explain it, you need to know something about the way your butt is built.

CHAPTER THREE

Why It Feels Like You're Being Impaled By A Fence Post.

It isn't just your sphincter causing all that pain; it's your "S-curve" as well as involuntary puborectal contractions. Discover your anatomical structure so you can make The Sexhalation Method work better.

RELAXING YOUR SPHINCTER during anal sex will go a long way to eliminating pain, but it only gets you so far into the promised land. There are two other points of pain to watch out for. In order to prevent them from doing the devil's work you have to understand a bit of butt anatomy. Let's start with something that might surprise you.

You Have Two Sphincters.

You may only have one anus but two connecting sphincters surround it. They are distinct but overlapping bands of muscle tissue. And while they serve the exact same function (regulating grand openings and final close-outs) they go about it in different ways. You are most familiar with the external sphincter because you can order it to tighten and release. Here, try it. Squinch your starfish by using the muscles to stop yourself from peeing. Got it? Tighten, release, tighten, release. Now, this time with feeling! Tighten, release. Now do five fast tightens. Get it? You can boss that part of your butt around. Feel like taking a crap but there's no bathroom around? No problem. You can will your external sphincter not to open. At least for a while.

But the internal sphincter? You can't tell it to do shit. And I mean that in every sense of the word. You are not its boss. Like your blood pressure and heartbeat, you cannot directly control it.

Do this: Put your hands in front of you as if you're praying. Now intertwine your fingers down to the webbing and press your palms together as tight as you can. Now keep everything connected and completely relax both hands. Notice the small opening between the side of your thumb and your index finger? This is the opening to your anus. If somebody tried to poke their finger through that opening it would feel snug but it'd go in pretty easy.

Now tighten both hands as hard as you can. The left hand is the internal sphincter you cannot directly control. The right hand is the external sphincter you can. Keeping the left hand tight as a drum, completely relax your right hand. Your right hand (external sphincter) is relaxed so a *slight* opening was created. But your left hand (internal sphincter) is so tight that it won't let a poking finger through very easily.

Welcome to bottoming's first dilemma: The left hand doesn't know what the right hand is doing. Or more accurately, the left hand doesn't *care* what the right hand is doing. The internal and external sphincter can and often do work independently of each other. In order to make penetration smooth and effortless *both* sphincters have to get on the same page. In the next chapter, you're going to learn how to do that, but first, let's talk about another pain in the ass. Did you know that...

You Own A Sling?

It's way down deep in your dungeon where it belongs. The puborectal sling is a strong ring of supportive muscle that creates a curve in the rectum. You're not the only thing that isn't straight in your house, you know. Neither is your rectum. The sling pulls the lower end of the rectum toward your belly button before it straightens out to eventually become the anal canal, which is the passageway from your sphincter to the rectum.

This is important to know because the S curve caused by the sling is responsible for pain point #2. The more the sling pulls the lower rectum toward the navel, the more pronounced your S curve will be. Why would that create pain? Because unless you find a way to straighten the S curve your partner's penis will ram the rectal wall at up to ninety degrees and make you think you're getting stabbed on the inside with a bat. Raise your left hand, palm down. Now poke the palm with your right index finger. This is the penis hitting the rectal wall caused by the S curve. Now move your palm up to ninety degrees (as if you were shaking somebody's hand) and poke it with your index finger the way you did before. You can't. Your finger glides up your palm. That's what bottoming will feel like if you straighten out your S curve.

Now, there is a third point of pain. It's located across the entire puborectal region, and it's caused by a simple law of nature.

Your Body Automatically Contracts When You Insert Something Into It.

The puborectal region is not used to being penetrated. It will interpret the penetrating object as an invading army that must be repelled. Never mind the sphincter and the sling (sounds like a new Disney fairy tale, doesn't it? *"The Sphincter & The Sling"*). Wait. Where was I? Oh, yes, all the muscles, fibers and tissues in the area will contract when you insert a foreign object and make it exceedingly difficult to bottom. These contractions are simply the body trying to protect itself. We'll talk later about how to neutralize this natural reaction, but for now...

Let's Review.

You have three potential points of pain:

1. The Internal And External Sphincters.

They work together (and apart) to keep things in or out. Sometimes they work inde-pendently of each other, which is a bummer because it makes complete relaxation a bit trickier. Think of your hands clasped together tightly. If one hand loosens but the other doesn't, it's harder to get a finger through the hole. If both hands loosen the finger slides in easily. It's fairly easy to relax your external sphincter because it obeys conscious command. The internal sphincter? Not so much. Your challenge is to relax *both* sphincters so that a penis can get through them without causing pain.

2. The S Curve Caused By The Puborectal Sling.

Even if you get past the gatekeeping sphincters, you have to deal with the S curve in your rectum caused by the puborectal sling. It forces the lower end of the rectum to curve toward the navel, thus creating a situation where the incoming penis hits the anal wall almost perpendicularly. The pain will make you wish impotence on your partner. Think of a highway guardrail curving into the middle of the road. Less road and more guardrail means the car is bound to hit the barrier and cause some damage.

3. The Puborectal Contractions.

The body knows that the best way to repel an invading force is to shut everything down tightly. Because the puborectal region is only used to things going out of it, the attempt to put something into it is going to be met with withering skepticism. Muscles in the surrounding area will clamp down hard and make you pay dearly for your impertinence.

These are the three pain points that made you stop bottoming when you tried or *will* stop you if you attempt to bottom without having a strategy that addresses them. Fortunately, we are about to do that.

CHAPTER FOUR

How Porn Star Bottoms
Relax Their Sphincters.

Not all do it, or need to, but the ones that do swear by it.
Find out whether you should use their controversial method.

THEIR SECRET IS PRETTY PUBLIC, ACTUALLY. It's just that you will never see it onscreen. A great deal of porn star bottoms sniff poppers to relax their sphincters. There's a lot to be said for poppers, but there's a lot to be said against them, too.

Let's start from the top. What are poppers? They're a liquid made from the alkyl nitrite family. Most commonly it's slang for amyl nitrate (AM-il NYE-trite), but it's also known as amyl, butyl, and isobutyl nitrite. In prescription form it's used by inhalation to relieve the pain of angina attacks. It works by relaxing blood vessels and increasing the supply of blood and oxygen to the heart. There was a popping sound when you crushed the cloth-covered glass capsules they used to come in, hence the darling name.

"Poppers" as a recreational drug are illegal, but they're sold legally by a sleight of hand—they're marketed as air fresheners, video head cleaners, leather cleaners or even nail polish remover. You'll also see them referred to as 'aromas,' 'liquid incense' and by brand names like Liquid Gold and Rush.

How Poppers Work To Loosen Your Sphincter.

Right before intercourse, porn stars sniff the fumes in a bottle of poppers, all off-camera. Within seconds, chemicals in the fumes cause blood vessels to dilate, which drops blood pressure and increases heart rate. *"There's a rush of blood to your head,"* one porn star said, *"Your heart beats fast and all your muscles relax."* Especially, the sphincter muscles. Most people who use poppers feel an excited, light-headed feeling for 1-2 minutes before the effects wear off.

Porn stars use poppers because they work. They really will loosen your sphincter. They'll also lower your inhibitions. But like all drugs, the downsides are enormous and you'd be a fool not to consider them.

Poppers Are The Main Reason Porn Star Bottoms Don't Get Hard.

Poppers are a perfect example of the law of unintended consequences. Yes, they loosen the sphincter but they relax *all* muscles in the body. Including the muscles that support erections. One of the main side effects of poppers is impotence. In fact, when porn star bottoms want another sniff of the poppers during anal sex, the top often has to turn away so he doesn't breathe in the fumes and lose his erection.

I'm guessing you're not looking to lose your hardon when you bottom, so that's a giant red flag if you're considering using poppers. Now, not everybody loses their erection but enough do to warrant a good hard think before you use them.

Do Poppers Cause HIV?

Absolutely not, but studies show they might play a big role in getting HIV passed on if you're not conscious of how they can affect your body and most importantly, your behavior. Examples:

- Poppers expand blood vessels everywhere, including the lining of your rectum, increasing the chances that you'll bleed.

- Poppers can affect your judgment, leaving your senses, as well as the unused condom, on the floor.

- Because poppers really do relax the sphincter, you might be tempted to have rough sex, which increases the chance of internal bleeding.

- Poppers temporarily make the immune system weaker, leaving you more open to infection.

Do the math. Increased chance of internal bleeding + cloudy judgment leading to no condom/rough sex + weaker immune system = High likelihood of HIV transmission. If you ask an HIV expert to describe the most likely scenario of an infection, it would go something like this: "When an HIV negative man uses poppers while bottoming for an HIV positive guy who doesn't use condoms."

But Wait, There's More Bad News.

What, that's not enough? Hey, don't confuse the message with the messenger. There are a few other things you should know about poppers. The most common side effects are headaches and dizziness (sometimes immediately). Some people faint, which makes sense because poppers dramatically lower blood pressure. It's the main reason you should NEVER use poppers if you're taking Viagra, Cialis or Levitra. All of these drugs lower blood pressure. Combining them is a great way to risk death.

Poppers aren't addictive but they can be habit-forming. Plus, the more you use them the less effect they have, so you have to keep sniffing more and more to get the same effect.

Should You Use Poppers?

I'm not your mother. Or your doctor. It's up to you. I just want to make sure you have all the facts before making a decision. Under the right conditions they might make sense for you. People are people and there's bound to be curiosity about doing what so many porn stars do to bottom without pain, so as a public service I want to introduce you to…

The Intelligent Way Of Using Poppers.

In the spirit of making sure that curiosity doesn't kill the cat, I've outlined the safest way for you to use poppers. Let me be clear, I am not advising you to use poppers. I am advising that if YOU decide to use them, that you put some thought into how. I spoke to several drug experts and here's what they consider an intelligent approach to using poppers:

- Do not use poppers if you take drugs or supplements that lower blood pressure. This is especially true of erectile dysfunction drugs like Viagra or supplements like Yohimbe.

- Do not use poppers if you have low or high blood pressure, a heart condition or glaucoma or are using medications to treat these conditions.

- Do not use poppers if you're using other recreational drugs like ecstasy, speed, cocaine or crystal meth. They all put strain on your heart.

- Only sniff the fumes. Keep the liquid in the bottle. You will get a chemical burn on your skin if you spill it. It's easy to spill it with lubed-up fingers, so be careful! Wash off with water if you do spill it. God help you if you get it in your eyes. Call 911 immediately.

- Never, ever swallow the chemicals in the bottle.

- Keep poppers away from cigarettes, candles and lighters. They are extremely flammable.

- Avoid forcing air into a stuffed nose. The chemicals can cause ear and sinus infections.

◆ Use the dose doctors recommend for their angina patients: Pass it back and forth close to your nose and inhale the vapor several (1-6) times.

◆ Use the repeat dosage strategy doctors recommend for their angina patients: Repeat within 1-5 minutes. Do not exceed a total of 2 doses in a 10-minute period. Again, for the intellectually feeble, let me repeat that: *Do not exceed a total of 2 doses in a 10-minute period.*

Just Say Know.

Let's talk a little more about drug use because as you'll see in the next chapters, porn star bottoms don't stop at poppers. They're using everything they can get their hands on. So this is probably a good time for me to articulate a rather nuanced view of taking recreational drugs. Over the years I've received some remarkably moving, sometimes enraging but mostly entertaining emails from readers about drug use in the gay community. I offer these provocative emails—and my answers to them—as a way of getting you to think critically about your own decisions to use or not use drugs. I leave the choice of using drugs up to you. The only thing I insist on is that if you do choose to use them, that you use them intelligently. "Just Say No" is a valid response. But so is "Just Say Know."

Hey, Woody!

You're the only one I can turn to because I'm too scared to ask anybody I know. Last month my 24-year-old boyfriend died while I was fucking him. He sniffed some poppers and suddenly lost consciousness. I panicked. I called 911. The emergency workers burst in asking "Is he on any kind of drugs?"

In my panic I said "No." I was too scared. You see, I got the poppers illegally from a hospital I work at. I figured if I told the truth there would be an investigation and they'd find out. None of my friends who've "fallen out" at parties ever died, so I figured my boyfriend would be okay.

He died en route to the hospital. The autopsy report said the cause of death was unknown, but I think he died because I didn't tell the emergency team he was on drugs. I'm haunted by what I've done– I can't sleep at night, I have trouble eating. I'm too ashamed to go to a therapist. I need a safe, anonymous person so I'm turning to you. Would the emergency workers have done anything differently, could they have saved my boyfriend's life, if I had told them he was using poppers?

– Haunted in Texas

Dear Haunted:

This story is so shocking that when I convened my panel of experts they practically gasped. But to a person (including an EMT—Emergency Medical Technician) they all agreed that emergency workers on the scene would have done nothing differently had they known about the use of poppers.

The only way the information would have been useful is if it were possible to pump poppers out of his system or if there were an "antidote" for it. There isn't.

Poppers open up your veins and coronary arteries by relaxing the muscles in these vessels. They often plunge blood pressure to dangerously low levels. The EMTs already knew he was in shock because monitoring blood pressure is standard procedure.

The consensus of my panel is that your boyfriend died from unsustainable low blood pressure brought on by the poppers. But there were contributing factors: Anal intercourse stimulates the vagal nerve, which drops blood pressure and slows the pulse. Also, your boyfriend may have had arrythmia (a change in the regular beat of the heart). This common condition could have accelerated the drop in blood pressure.

You didn't kill your boyfriend. He was an adult of sound mind and body who asked you for the drugs he took. Still, you have to face the moral implications of giving someone you loved the agent of their death. It was a horrible accident of chance, but there is no getting around the fact that you contributed to it.

You have to find a way to release the guilt and secrecy haunting you and create meaning out of this tragedy. Find a therapist you trust and work it out with him. You have some work to do, starting with his family. When you're emotionally strong enough, let them know about the poppers (but not how you got them—it's irrelevant). You owe them that.

You owe your boyfriend, too. You owe him the possibility that some good can come out of this tragedy. Like stopping it from happening to someone else. Devote yourself to helping people make sound drug choices.

For some it'll be to never use them; for others to use them judiciously. In the memory of your boyfriend, find a way to forgive yourself so you can make a difference in someone's life.

Hey, Woody!

Your advice to people about using poppers SUCKED. What the fuck is "intelligent use of poppers?" There is no such thing as an intelligent use of poppers. Why don't you wake up, fool? How about telling people not to use them at all, like any responsible expert would? Well, you're no expert and you're certainly not responsible with that kind of advice. Poppers damage the heart and fuck up the immune system. I can't believe you'd write an article telling people how to use them. Shame on you, Woody. I've read the last of you.

– An ex-reader

Dear ex-:

First of all, you must be confusing me with Ann Landers. She's the one who gives the kind of dried-vagina advice you're looking for.

My advice is not directed at children, but at grown adults, the kind who've already made up their minds about whether they're going to use drugs. I have never advocated nor condemned drug use. My role is to haul out the Stupid Meter and call the crowd's attention to it when it goes off. And goddammit does it goes off in the gay community.

It's a good thing the Stupid Meter doesn't run on batteries—I'd be on a first-name basis with the Radio Shack cashier.

Do I think people should do drugs? No. Do I think they shouldn't do drugs? No. I think people should make their own decisions and people like you and me should stay out of it.

We should have the same penalties for drug abuse as we do for alcohol abuse. Namely, if you're not hurting people or property, we should leave you the hell alone.

Do something stupid, like Driving Under the Influence, and you should have the book thrown at you. Along with the vase, picture frames and whatever else was on the shelf with the book.

We're exposed to alcohol education all the time (Budweiser "Drink Responsibly" ads come to mind), but you think we shouldn't be exposed to drug education?

No matter what the penalty, there are three things that men will always play with: Fire, drugs and themselves. And not necessarily in that order. The "Just Say No" mentality was given its chance and it failed spectacularly. Your corner is always yapping about giving it more time, and maybe you're right; maybe we should give it another shot—after all we only gave it a hundred and forty fucking years to work. Maybe that's just not enough time to see results.

Hey, Woody!

After 30 hours with no sleep, which included 2 nights of dancing, drinking, using Ecstasy and "G", someone slipped me an overdose of this new thing called Liquid X.

In about an hour I was so messed up I couldn't complete a sentence. Before long I was vomiting. But not just vomiting, I mean VOMITTING. As in the medic said I almost drowned in it.

Within another hour I was in a coma unable to breathe for myself. The medics took me to the local hospital and put me in the ICU (Intensive Care Unit). The doctors told my friends there was a good chance a vessel busted in my brain and I may have incurred brain damage and/or possible brain death. They said the next 6 to 12 hours would be critical. Of course, I have no memories of all this.

About six hours into a coma, I found my way back into consciousness and I was horrified at what I saw: A tube was down my throat breathing for me. I was con-nected to all kinds of wires and other not so pleasant things like a catheter jammed up my dick to siphon the urine out.

It's a miracle that within 48 hours of being taken into the hospital in a coma, be-ing kept alive by a machine, I walked out on my own two feet. But unfortunately, right into PTSD (Post Traumatic Stress Disorder). I can't sleep and when I do, I have nightmares that I'm choking. My doc has given me Ambien to sleep and Clonipin to calm me down, which has helped a lot.

For a few weeks, I cried all the time, though that's getting better too. I've been a party boy for a while now and needless to say, this near-death experience has changed that part of my life completely. I don't touch the stuff anymore and I'm telling everyone to stay away from it.

Woody, would you print this letter and tell everyone to flush all their drugs down the toilet? Everyone I know in the scene reads your column. Do the responsible thing and tell them to stay off drugs.

– Over it

Dear Over it:

You must have me confused with Ann Landers. I don't give dried-vagina advice.

I will never tell people to stop doing drugs unless it's idiots like you taking them. Our thirst for adventure can't, and shouldn't be quashed.

You made an awful mistake and now you want everyone else to pay for it. I'm not buying it. Most people who take drugs do it responsibly. You didn't. You fell off the stupid tree and hit every branch on the way down.

I know you're hurting and you genuinely want to help your friends avoid what you went through. But you're never going to do it by becoming a pain-in-the-ass moralist.

Get therapy. You need to find out how can you use this awful experience, this journey into darkness, into something that will help you and the people around you.

I have a vested interest in keeping you guys alive. If you keep dying book sales will go down and out comes my stumbling drunk of an editor demanding I give back my royalties. And if that happens believe me, it'll be ME spiking your water with liquid X.

Look, throughout time people have taken drugs and they're never going to stop. The best advice I ever heard on drugs came from Sister Kitty Catalyst of the Sisters of Perpetual Indulgence: "There's nothing fabulous about a trip to the emergency room. The lighting is bad, the outfits are horrid, and they have no idea what a VIP line is."

Amen, sister.

Hey Woody!

You moron, I can't believe you said "I will never tell people to stop doing drugs." How can you endorse using something dangerous enough to kill you or put you in a coma?

I'm an agnostic on the question of whether people should use drugs. I think people should make up their own minds. You think that my unwillingness to condemn drug use is tantamount to advocating it. You're wrong.

Hey Woody!

I've never been more disgusted than reading your flippant answer to the guy who almost died of an overdose. He deserved your sympathy, not your lame jokes.

I don't do sympathy in this column, asshole. In the dictionary sympathy rests between Shit and Syphilis. That guy didn't need my pity, he needed my support, both for processing the horrible event that almost took his life and to find a meaningful way to stop people from dying or becoming vegetables. He was on track on the first issue, off-track on the second.

Hey Woody!

How could you call a guy who almost died of an overdose a "pain in the ass moralist" because he's trying to get people to stop using drugs? You suck.

Because pain-in-the-ass moralists make things worse. They're the reasons drugs are illegal, which means they're not regulated like alcohol or nicotine, which means people don't really know what they're taking, which exponentially increases the chance of overdosing.

Pain-in-the-ass moralists came up with teaching abstinence in high schools and what did we get? The highest rate of teenage pregnancies in the world.

Pain-in-the-ass moralists gave us Prohibition and what did we get? Increased consumption of hard liquor.

Policies based on moral outrage produce massive failure. If the guy really wants to help people he'd replace his pious Just Say No campaign with a hard-boiled Just Say Know approach. If we get people to Know their limits, Know the dangers, and Know when to stop, we could actually prevent a lot of needless deaths and injuries.

Hey Woody!

Would you ever say "I will never tell people to stop having unsafe sex?" Then why would you say it about drugs?

Would you really expect me to discourage people from having sex because sex is dangerous? Or would you expect me to preach safety, to use a condom, to be responsible? Why should drugs be any different?

Hey Woody!

Drugs are *illegal*. I think it's immoral to advocate any kind of use, responsible or not, for something you can get arrested for.

You pinhead. Homosexuality is illegal too. Check your state's criminal laws and see what they say about sodomy. By your definition I'm being immoral every time I tell you to use a condom.

Hey Woody!

There is no such thing as "responsible" drug use. You might as well teach pyromaniacs how to light a house on fire in a way that won't harm the building.

Bullshit. Drugs are not in and of themselves dangerous. It's the way you use them that makes them so. Drugs are like electricity. They can electrocute you or light your house, depending on whether you apply stupidity or intelligence to it.

Hey Woody!

You are a mean, evil queen who doesn't care that our gay brothers are killing themselves.

And you're a hand-wringing schoolmarm addicted to the ecstasy of sanctimony. You care more about making people wrong than about reducing injuries.

I spend a lot of time writing about responsible drug use because I'm alarmed at what gay men are doing to themselves. I don't have to do that, you know. Last time I looked this was a sex advice column not a drug education class.

Hey Woody!

How can you make "clear-headed" decisions if you're on a substance that clouds your judgment?

The same way you make responsible judgments when your dick is hard. The same way you make them when you drink. One stroke, one drink, one bump, one hit at a time.

You make responsible decisions BEFORE your judgment is clouded. Sorry, but a hit of ecstasy or a snort of Tina does not automatically cloud most people's judgment (if it does, then halve your first hit).

It IS true that the more drugs (or alcohol) you take the less rational your judgment becomes. The trick is to start slow and constantly ask yourself this question:

"Can I have one more hit and still stay in control?"

Hey Woody!

You're acting as if "control" is that easy with drugs. You forget they're highly addictive.

Compared to what? According to the U.S. Food & Drug Administration, about 8% of people who drink alcohol are dependent. The FDA did not break out club drugs, but experts believe about 12% of people who use club drugs are dependent. This means about 88% of people who do club drugs don't get addicted.

Now what was your point?

Here's the rest of the FDA's breakout of a drug's users who are dependent: Hallucinogens 9%, marijuana 12%, cocaine 21%.

Nicotine is the drug that has the highest percentage of dependency among its users (80%). My guess is you were smoking a cigarette while you typed your outrage over drug addiction.

Hey, Woody!

I'm with you. It seems to me that the more shrill the warnings become about using drugs the more people want to do them.

Ever heard of "The Romeo and Juliet Effect?" Romeo Montague and Juliet Capulet came from feuding families. They fell deeply in love, despite fierce parental opposition, and ended up in a double-suicide.

Gee, I wonder what would have happened if their parents had paid no attention?

A lot of psychologists believe they would have broken up. A team of shrinks did a study of 140 teenage relationships. Here's what they found: Those couples who had interfering parents felt greater love for each other and expressed a higher desire to get married.

If parental interference decreased researchers noticed that romantic feelings cooled at a corresponding rate.

What's all this got to do with drugs? That which is forbidden is desired more greatly.

Hey, Woody!

Is it possible that all your lofty speeches about using responsibly are about justifying your own drug use, maybe even a drug problem? You've always been honest, don't stop now.

I'm not ashamed to say that I've had my share of problems with drugs. At one point in my life I couldn't go a day without giving myself a fix. My head would start to pound, my hands would start to tremble and I couldn't really concentrate without it.

But enough about my morning coffee.

Here's my club drug history: I've had great experiences that make me understand why people take them and I've had terrible experiences that make me understand why people stop. At this point, I only do them at huge party events, maybe once every couple of months.

Hey, Woody!

Do you really believe that drugs aren't more harmful than alcohol?

No, I believe drugs are more harmful.

Go from one cigarette to thirty in a night and you'll get sick. Go from one drink to ten and you'll pass out. Go from one hit of G to two and you might die.

So yes, drugs are more dangerous. Which is why, if you're going to use them, you have to be even more responsible than when you use alcohol.

Hey, Woody!

I'm totally into the scene but I have to admit things are starting to get a little out

of hand. One of my friends actually died from a crystal addiction and several oth-ers landed in the ER. I'm in control when I do drugs and I try to get my friends to ease up a little on the throttle, but sometimes they go too far. Last week a friend fell out. As we were waiting outside none of us knew what to do for him (he was passed out). I know this isn't a sex question but what are you supposed to do while you wait for the ambulance?

– The Helper

Dear Helper:

What should you do while you wait for the ambulance? Another bump. Never let the selfish flailing of a dying friend get in the way of a good buzz.

Seriously, I have to compliment you on the intelligent way you're using drugs and for the compassion you've shown your friend by sticking with him till help arrived.

But enough complimenting—it ruins my reputation. Here's what you should do when He's-Ruining-It-For-The-Rest-of-Us bites off a little more than he should snort:

1) **Keep him breathing**. If he isn't, then do mouth-to-cock resuscitation. Put his mouth on your cock and blow. It's always the first thing I do when a cute guy falls out. It doesn't do him any good but it makes me feel blissful, loving and spiritually connected to the brotherhood of man, and isn't that what the scene's all about?

If he isn't cute, or if you've already had him, then do mouth-to-mouth breathing. Make sure he doesn't aspirate any vomitus if he upchucks (damn, why can't my medical advisors just say "Make sure he doesn't swallow chunks of his own vomit?" They're always trying to impress me with big words). Anyway, getting vomit chunks in your lungs can cause pneumonia and kill you, no lie, within three days. That's why surgeons don't perform operations for at least 12-24 hours after you've eaten.

2) **Check head-to-toe for unseen injuries.** You're looking for fractures, head injuries, etc. Femur fractures (breaks in the thighbone) can kill because they bleed so much and so quickly. So be sure to check the upper inside thigh. Relieve him of any drugs he's carrying. Consider it your reward for being so helpful. If a neck injury is suspected, stabilize the head, neck and body. Don't twist or turn it, unless it's to steal his money when nobody's looking. Try to

keep him immobilized until you've gone through all his pockets and be sure to check the inside of his socks. I always find an extra $20 bill there.

3) **Do what the EMS workers say.** Answer their questions truthfully—tell them what drugs your friend was taking. The emergency team isn't interested (nor does it have the authority) to arrest you, so don't cop out on your responsibility to help. Don't tell them you went through his pockets and filched all the valuables, though. Those EMS vultures hate competition and they're liable to strap you onto the gurney just out of spite.

Once they load your friend onto the ambulance the EMTs will give him some combination of oxygen, heparin (prevents blood clotting) and fluids. Keeping victims breathing is the biggest challenge of any overdose situation. Especially when I'm in the ambulance throttling the victims for being so goddamn stupid.

You know, most people start anti-drug campaigns after seeing some of the tragic consequences of drug abuse. I'm more realistic. I start anti-stupidity campaigns. In fact, my slogan is "Just Say Know." If you're going to party, Know what you're taking, Know your limits, Know what combinations to avoid.

If you can't stay in control do us all a favor and stay home. Ambulances should be chasing heart-attack victims, not idiots who can't use drugs responsibly.

Hey, Woody!

My pothead boyfriend smokes at least every other day and he's got zero interest in sex. He puts the lack in slacker. The only thing standing upright in my house is the vacuum cleaner. Would it help if I slipped him some Viagra? Is it safe for him to take the big blue pill while he's stoned? He just doesn't seem to want me or anyone else for that matter.

– Begging for it

Dear Begging:

I'm still trying to figure out how you "slip" Viagra into somebody. Like Tang, I guess you could crush it into a powder and mix it with water. But then we'd have to call it Bang.

There are no known interactions between Viagra and pot; as long as he doesn't have any blood pressure or heart conditions he shouldn't have any problems. But I doubt it'll do any good. Viagra can give you a boner but it can't give you what comes before it—desire.

Sexual arousal starts above the belt, not below it. Brain cells get activated, which start the blood flow to you-know-where. If brain cells can't process a sexually-exciting image (say, you in "Dance Fever" leotards) because there's enough marijuana haze to make asthmatics long for the cleanliness of Los Angeles air, then what good is Viagra going to do?

A lot of scientists believe marijuana decreases testosterone, sperm count and consequently, sexual desire. It's been proven in laboratory rats that marijuana changes the chemistry of the nerve cells in the brain affecting sexual behavior, the same cells that regulate hormones producing testosterone and sperm.

But rats, schmats, nobody really knows marijuana's sexual effects on humans. The limited research is contradictory. Some studies show decreases in testosterone and sperm count; some don't.

The studies may be contradictory but don't be a fool. You can't do anything in excess and not have it affect your sex life. I'm afraid you're going to have to give your boyfriend something harsher than Viagra—an ultimatum. It's decision time: Your ass or his pot. Maybe he needs an unbiased source for a decision. Send a naked picture of yourself and a sample of his stash and let me be the judge.

Hey, Woody!

Get the splinter out of your ass! Your lack of any warning to the potential harm of meth and other drugs pisses me off. For too long the "gay mainstream" has placed the discussion of drug use in the closet in fear of stepping into judgment. Mister Miller, because you are in a publication that is in the public domain, you have a responsibility to inform your readership. You affirmed drug use by not responding to its potential harm. You seem to be an angry and self-righteous man. If you step back and set aside your ego you may find the flaw in your work. We all like sex and lots of it. But the more chances we take with drugs the less experience we will have.

Your column is filled with half answered advice and potentially harmful statements. If you are not qualified to give advice, don't. You will do more harm than good. You must be informed to inform. If "need wood?" is an advice column give good advice. Otherwise place it in the editorial section.

—Spittin' Nails at your Tales

Dear Spit:

Yours is the kind of hypocrisy shared by society in general—that it's okay to alter your mood with alcohol but not with drugs. You conveniently took my statement out of context. I said, and I quote, *"I see nothing wrong with getting high on meth, just like I see nothing wrong with getting drunk on alcohol, as long as you're safe."* I stand by that statement.

Like most hypocritical windbag moralists railing about drug use, you probably typed out your letter while drinking a beer. According to your line of thinking, it's okay to numb your senses with wine, but not with K; it's okay to get wired with caffeine but not cocaine. I defy anyone to tell me the difference between a shot of tequila gold and a snort of crystal meth, other than its intensity and duration.

Compared to alcoholism, drug addiction is a pimple in the ass of substance abuse. According to every shrink's bible, the DSM-V (Diagnostic and Statistical Manual of Mental Disorders), approximately 35 million people have suffered alcohol dependence some time in their life. Know what it is for amphetamine dependence? About 2 million.

In the last six months, alcohol has probably been responsible for more deaths, divorces, and job loss than drugs have for the last 10 years. When men get infected by HIV because they exercised poor judgment in bed, that judgment is far more likely to be impaired by alcohol than drugs. Yet not a word in your letter showed the least concern for alcohol's potential damage. Why is that?

I'll tell you why. Because you think people should use only the depressants and stimulants that you use. By attacking drugs and not alcohol you can get buzzed AND feel superior.

You're pretending that I'm defending drug abuse when I'm really advocating moderation in all mood-altering agents. I'm tired of being denied pleasure because there's a group of idiots who abuse that pleasure. And I'm especially tired of people like you, who think the best way of protecting these idiots is to deny access to the majority of us who are responsible users.

This may come as a surprise, Mother Teresa, but a lot of guys like to have a little buzz when they're going to have sex, me included. I don't see anything wrong with that. Where that buzz comes from—vodka, marijuana, caffeine, dirty underwear—is irrelevant. What's relevant is that you maintain control so that you don't end up making stupid decisions you'll later regret.

And the fact that most people CAN maintain control really pisses off people like you because it derails your drug Armageddon argument. Most people in the scene are not drug addicts, just like most guys at a bar are not alcoholics.

You have a valid point about the growing gay drug culture and I share that concern. But "DON'T" as the last word in advising people isn't the answer. Look how well it worked for alcohol (Prohibition), teen-age pregnancy, and in our own community, the rise of unsafe sex.

I will continue advocating common sense in whatever mood changers people use. I do not "recommend" drugs anymore than I recommend alcohol. What I "recommend" more than anything is staying in control.

CHAPTER FIVE

The Porn Star Method Of Eliminating Pain.

Three Words: Drugs, Drugs, DRUGS!
But There's A Better Way.

WHAT DO STUPID DRUG DEALERS SAY when they get pulled over by the cops? *"You're not going to check the trunk are you?"* Well, check out the trunks of porn star bottoms and you're going to think they're mules for Colombian drug lords. You cannot talk about the porn industry without talking about recreational drugs. Tops use it to keep themselves hard, bottoms use it to keep their butts open and everyone else uses them, well, let's say for morale.

Crystal meth and ecstasy are the drugs of choice. Many porn star bottoms "slam" it (street for injecting it with a hypodermic needle). Others put it up their butts while others do it the old-fashioned way and snort or swallow it. *"A lot of bottoms get soft when they're getting fucked,"* one porn star said. *"When I slam, my dick gets instantly hard but it takes me longer to come. Makes me passionate with the top and especially it's the best when it's a group setting."*

Words to live by.

This is how prevalent drug use is in the industry—when we asked one porn star how studios handle an actor having a problem with bottoming, this is was his response: *"There's been some that whine, but then we just get them high as hell, and then they don't care."*

More words to live by.

When we asked how straight guys bottom in gay porn, if there were special ways they prepared newbies, several directors gave the same response: *"Uhm, yeah, get them very high."* One famous director (the most famous of the bunch we interviewed) said this when asked how they loosen up a bottom who just can't take large cargo: *"Always get him high. Give him GHB or something."*

We're running out of words to live by.

There are so many things wrong with the way the porn industry approaches bottom-ing I don't know whether to list them alphabetically, numerically or categorically. By now, you should know that generally speaking, I am agnostic on whether you should use recreational drugs. But on the specific issue of bottoming I am a total atheist—I absolutely do not believe in using drugs to bottom. You need to learn how to avoid pain; not how to mask it. Pain is a signal that SOMETHING IS WRONG. It is a sig-nal that you are harming yourself. Drugs might protect you from pain but they don't protect you from the consequences of that pain—a ripped anal lining, burst blood vessels, and bruising in the anorectal area. And they certainly won't protect you from HIV at that point.

People who cannot feel pain ("congenital analgesia") are in mortal danger every day of their lives. They could sit on a hot stove and not know it until they smell the burn-ing tissue. It's the same concept with guys who are drugged out and cannot feel pain when they bottom. They don't know the harm they cause themselves until it's too late.

In addition, drugs won't 'train' your sphincter muscles to relax which is critical to pain-free bottoming. Meaning, your sphincter muscles are going to be just as tight the next time you bottom. And that's why porn star bottoms who take drugs have to keep taking them if they don't want to experience excruciating pain.

What About Topical Analgesics Like Anal-Eze?

It isn't just recreational drugs you should stay away from, it's *anything* that artificially numbs the pain. Topical anesthetics like Anal Eze or Oragel are bad ways to, er, get to the bottom of your problem. Or rather, the problem of being a bottom.

Why? *Because anything that masks pain is going to cause harm.* Besides, the anesthet-ics won't work. They don't penetrate far enough to relax the muscle. It's like using full sentences to seduce a party boy: Good luck.

If you really want to try topical anesthetics you'll need a prescription from a doctor because the over-the-counter crap doesn't work. And if you do manage to get a pre-scription, I'd love to see your insurer's reaction to the diagnosis. I mean, what's your doctor going to say to get the treatment approved? "Patient has trouble getting fucked in the ass?"

Topical agents like Anal Eze have some unintended consequences even for porn stars, which is why most of them don't use it. As one porn star bottom told us:

I was shooting a film for a weekend period, and the first night I had gotten ripped up by a top and I had to compensate for that by using a numbing cream like Oragel or something similar. But anyhow, I used it to numb my ass so I could keep on shooting that weekend and one of the tops (another top) was playing with my ass and was beating my hole with his cock and got some of the Oragel on it and it went soft because my "ass cream" numbed his cock. So when he pulled out, his dick was soft and numb. The whole thing was, the giggle was, that my ass was so tight that it had made his dick go numb.

One More Bird-Brained Porn Industry Technique To Stop Pain.

One porn star bottom told us of a technique many bottoms in the industry use to contain the pain—ice. Here's what he said:

"Personally for me, I did not use any drugs whatsoever. The closest thing that I would do for numbing myself up especially if I was going to take someone really large is to take a cube of ice. If you shove a cube of ice up your ass, it's so cold, it will numb the sphincter muscle to prepare taking that dick. It's a common practice."

There are so many levels of wrong to using this technique it's hard to know where to start. Maybe with the idea that you should never mask the pain because it's your body's way of saying STOP? Nah, I've said that too often. How about this? You can't freeze a muscle with an ice cube. Besides, the source of pain is the stretching of the anus; the only way to avoid pain from over-stretching is to help the sphincter muscles *relax*, which ice does not do.

A Highly Effective Alternative To Drugs.

There is a much better way to pain-free bottoming and it doesn't involve drugs at all. Before we get into it, let's start with the two words you've probably heard from partners who tried to top you...

"Relax! Relax!"

How many times have you heard that from your partner? Hell, how many times have you said it to yourself? Telling someone to relax without showing them how is counter-productive. It actually increases anxiety and tension because on top of not relaxing you feel like a failure for not being able to relax!

Tension is the main source of pain when it comes to bottoming. When an object is forcefully inserted into a tense, clenched, tightly wound, clamped down set of muscles and tissue, it will damage, tear and bruise the area. But if the area is completely relaxed, an incoming object meets little to no resistance and slides in easily and without pain.

But how do you go from clenched and clamped to calm and relaxed? Think nice thoughts? Distract yourself? Count to ten? Breathe? How? Most of us do not have any idea how to calm ourselves to the point of complete relaxation, especially when we're experiencing stress. And if you want to experience stress all you have to do is look at the size of your partner's penis and then the size of your anus!

You don't need to be told to relax. You know that. If it were easy to relax while a large object the size of a penis goes into a tiny orifice the size of your anus you'd have already done it. One major reason you've failed is that a great deal of the puborectal region, like the internal sphincter, does not respond to conscious attempts at relaxation. What you need is a disciplined approach that shows you how to relax muscles that won't listen to you.

And that's why I'd like to introduce you to…

The Sexhalation Method

It's a systematic approach that completely relaxes rectal muscles that are both in and out of your conscious control. You will be able to relax muscles that listen to you (example: the external sphincter) as well as those that don't (example: the internal sphincter). It blends the proven concept of systematic desensitization with progressive muscle relaxation, pattern breathing and sexual imagery. Used correctly, The Sexhalation Method is guaranteed to eliminate all pain from anal sex. Not some. *All*. I developed this system with the help of a team of experts including a yoga guru, an expert in respiratory psychophysiology, and specialists in colo-rectal anatomy.

The Sexhalation Method is actually quite simple but it requires you to understand a few things about your body. Let's start by examining why so much of your butt tension is (seemingly) beyond your ability to control it. Do this: Tighten your sphincter as hard as you can right now for a count of five seconds. Notice how clamped down it feels. Now relax. Feels like you controlled your sphincter, no?

That's a trick question, because as you already know, you have two sphincter muscles, not one. The whole time you were clamping down on your external sphincter your internal sphincter was chillin' on the couch, sipping a cosmo, blithely unaware that its twin brother was being throttled. The external sphincter does not re-spond to your commands because like your heart beat, it's governed by the autonom-ic nervous system.

You can't make your heart beat faster by telling it to hurry up, but you can do things that result in a faster heartbeat (like pushups). We're going to use this same concept with your internal sphincter, as well as that other involuntary pain point—the puborectal sling. You can't will them to relax but you can do things that will result in relaxation. The first step in that direction is...

A Sexercise Plan For Your Sphincter.

The best way to consciously relax your external sphincter is, oddly enough, to tighten it. That's because the first step to relaxation is awareness of its opposite—tension. This is a key concept to bottoming without pain: Your sphincter will relax more if you make an effort to tense it first.

"Kegels" are exercises that will help you achieve this tension/relaxation dynamic. They will not only help your sphincter relax, they'll also make your erections harder, give you more control of your ejaculations and deliver more powerful orgasms. Named after the doctor that discovered the benefits of exercising the pubogenital muscles, Kegels don't just stimulate the sphincter muscles, but everything around them—the anal canal, the rectum, the prostate, and the puborectal sling. They'll make you more aware of your body and give you more control over the levers of re-laxation. Before I show you how to do them, let's review what we know about your sphincter "twins."

Your anus has two ring-like muscles that overlap and function independently of each other. The external sphincter is closest to the anal opening and with just a little conscious effort you can tense or relax it whenever you want. Because the external sphincter responds to conscious thought, you don't really need instructions on how to relax it. But you do need to tone it so that it can loosen more fully, and the best way to do that is to do Kegels. Here are the steps:

Step 1: Find Your Kegel Muscles.

You know when you're in the shower with your partner and you pee on him while he's not looking? And then he notices and yells at you to stop so you squeeze the muscles that stop the flow of urine in mid-stream? That's them!

Step 2: Contract And Release.

Squeeze the muscles you use to stop peeing, then release. Do ten in a row, three times a day. Then gradually increase the number of contractions.

Step 3: Vary The Exercises.

Try 'The Flutter' (tighten and let go quickly) and the 'Pinch and Hold' (tighten and don't let go till you count to fifteen).

Step 4: Vary The Positions.

Start by sitting or standing but then try it while lying on your back or side or even while squatting. Different positions tone the muscle quicker.

Step 5: Add Weight Training.

Put a towel on your erect penis and do the contractions. You want bragging rights? Do them with wet towels.

Step 6: Do Them When You're Hard.

Squeezing the PC muscles when you get an erection makes your penis jerk up. Hold a finger about an inch above your penis and flex hard enough to touch it 10 times in a row. Or go for the bonus round by placing your partner's mouth an inch away. Now *that's* what I call home fitness training.

The cool thing about "Kegels" is that you can do them anywhere—driving, walking, watching TV, doing dishes, or knitting a doily. No one will ever know. About the exercises I mean, not the knitting. Don't expect overnight success. While it should only take a couple of weeks to heighten the sphincter's relaxation response, it takes four to six weeks of *daily* exercise (aim for at least 100 contractions) to see the other benefits, like stronger erections and more intense ejaculations.

Kegels Will Help You Shoot Further.

Orgasms happen via a spinal cord reflex that causes strong rhythmic contractions in the urogenital system. Your ejaculation isn't ruled by your hand, your partner's mouth, or your wild imagination. It's ruled by the urethra, the prostate and the pubogenital muscles as they involuntarily contract. You can't do anything to strengthen the urethra or the prostate other than having frequent orgasms, but the puborectal muscles? Kegels can make them stronger, which in turn make orgasmic contractions more forceful, which then propel the semen out of the urethra faster.

An Interesting Aside:

Ever notice that most porn stars "shoot" rather than "dribble" when they ejaculate? All is not what it seems. To get the money shot they want, directors will often use synthetic semen, which is shot-squeezed from a small tube. The preferred substance is condensed milk.

Okay, enough asides. Hit the floor and give me a hundred Kegels!

Why Relaxing Your Internal Sphincter Is So Crucial To Pain-Free Bottoming.

Now that you're toning the puborectal muscles with Kegels, it's time to train our attention on the internal sphincter, which again, does not respond to conscious efforts at relaxation. It's critical to get this involuntary muscle to relax because if you don't, there is a high likelihood that intercourse will cause bleeding, putting you at major risk for HIV and other STD's.

Let me explain. Anal "pillows" are attached to the internal sphincter through connective tissue and muscle fibers. They inflate with blood to help prevent the brown stuff from coming out when you don't want it to. They also inflate with blood as an initial blocking reaction to something going in.

When these pillows partially drain they allow a smooth, healthy dump as well as the safe insertion of your favorite man or man-made object. But forcefully trying to insert an object through a tense internal sphincter ruptures these blood-filled anal pillows, and oh, dear, there goes the sheets. It isn't just sex that ruptures the anal pillows —it's also straining on the toilet. In fact, if you see blood in the toilet water or on toilet paper when you wipe, it's a safe bet you ruptured the anal pillows.

The only way to make sure blood drains from these pillows is to relax the internal sphincter. If the internal sphincter is not relaxed, the anal cushions congest with blood. When something is forced out you get hemorrhoids (protrusions from the anal cushions) or fissures (tears or cracks in the anal lining). When something is forced in, well, red is a wonderful color on you, I'm sure.

The Four Pillars Of The Sexhalation Method.

Now that you have a little butt background, you're almost ready to test-drive The Sexhalation Method. But first, let's talk a little about the four pillars that make it work:

1.   **Systematic Desensitization.**

Tension equals pain. Relaxation provides pleasure. Doing your Kegels will build the foundation of the relaxation response—a supple, toned external sphincter that obeys on command. While that helps the entire pubogenital area, we have to pay special attention to your *internal* sphincter. We must train it to perceive the insertion of a finger, toy or penis as a sign of desirability not danger. The Sexhalation Method will do this through a process called systematic desensitization, a scientifically proven way to decrease tension and increase relaxation. Systematic desensitization is a way of *gradually* conditioning your body to accept certain sensations without experiencing pain. Notice the emphasis on the word *gradual.* For example, if you want to use your finger to explore yourself, systematic desensitization argues that you wouldn't pitch your finger through your sphincter like a toilet plunge (ouch!). Instead, you insert it an eighth of an inch, wait until all sensations disappear, go in another eighth of an inch, wait, then go another eighth of an inch until before you know it you've inserted half of the Eiffel Tower in your rectum without a single painful moment!

2.   **Pattern Breathing.**

The second pillar of The Sexhalation Method is rhythmic breathing. Breath isn't just the cornerstone of relaxation, but the foundation of life. It's the first thing you do when you're born and the last thing you do when you die. When you're stressed (like, oh, I don't know, expecting excruciating pain during anal intercourse) you will experience restricted and shallow breathing. The chest barely rises during inhalation, doesn't extend into the abdomen, and the exhalation is rarely complete. Shallow, fast breathing is a sign of muscle tension. It operates on a dual feedback loop: Tension causes shallow breathing, which causes more tension, which causes more shallow breathing.

Deep, slow breathing, on the other hand, is a sign of relaxation. It too operates on a feedback loop: Relaxation causes deep, slow breaths which causes more relaxation which causes more deep, slow breaths. Think about it: What is your breath like when you're anxious or fearful? Shallow and fast. What is your breath like when you first wake up? Deep and slow.

Notice your breathing when you're in a stressful situation and you'll come to understand something yoga masters have known for centuries:

Constricted breathing causes muscle tension.

Notice your breathing when you're relaxed and you'll come to understand the flip side of this observation:

Expanded breathing causes muscle relaxation.

The Sexhalation Method uses this concept of constriction/expansion to help you relax both sphincters. Here, take it for a test run: Inhale deeply and fully (through your nose) for a slow count of four. When you reach the end of the inhalation, pause for a full second. Now exhale for a slow count of six. When you reach the end of the exhale pause for a full second. Then inhale for a count of four and start the process again. Do this three and four times and you'll notice a subtle wave of relaxation extending throughout your body. If you don't feel it, don't worry, you will with practice. Pattern breathing won't just help with relaxing your sphincter muscles, it will help you release tension in every area of your life, whether it's waiting to get a flu shot or standing in line at the post office. Hey, come to think of it, both of those things resemble bottoming—they force you to deal with pricks!

3.   **Progressive Muscle Relaxation.**

The third pillar in The Sexhalation Method is the conscious and deliberate tightening and releasing of the sphincter muscles. As stated before, the best way to fully relax any muscle is to first tighten it as hard as you can before releasing it slowly. It's the law of opposites, like light and dark. You cannot fully know darkness until the sun hits your face and vice versa. Progressive muscle relaxation operates on the same basis. You can get muscles to relax more by first increasing the tension. When you release the tension there's a more dramatic experience of relaxation. Do this: Without moving, note the tension in your shoulders. Now physically try to relax the shoulders. Couldn't tell much difference, could you? Now, tense your shoulders by bringing them to your ears and hold it for thirty seconds. Now relax your shoulders. Do you see how much more noticeable the release of tension feels? We are going to use this concept, this law of opposites, on your rectal muscles and you're going to be amazed at the results.

4.   **Sexual Imagery**

The fourth pillar of The Sexhalation Method is erotic thought. The point to bottoming isn't to fill your orifice. It's to experience the presence of another man inside your body. It's to give yourself to another man, to surrender to the strength and hardness of his masculinity, to capitulate to the cock and it's mastery over you. This is an exciting thing that you should keep in mind while you do The Sexhalation Method. Desire is both the fuel and the point. Let it drive the proceedings. You *want* this. You're not practicing to get a flu shot—you're practicing to get a shot at sexual ecstasy. There's a big difference between relaxing for something painful and relaxing for something pleasurable. As you do these Sexhalation exercises bring up the most vivid images you can of your date/boyfriend/ husband/neighbor/porn star or whomever is floating your boat at the moment.

The Secret To Pain-Free Bottoming: The Sexhalation Method

The Sexhalation Method (let's shorten it to "Sexhalation") is a new approach to sexual insertion. As I mentioned before, I developed it with a team made up of a yoga guru, a psychologist specializing in respiratory psychophysiology, and colo-rectal specialists. Each member of the team contributed their fact-filled, field-tested views on relaxation theory, sexual response, anatomy, pleasure centers and pain points. Then we put it all together into a step-by-step system that all but guarantees a smooth bottoming experience. Sexhalation is the answer to a vexing question that stops millions of gay men from bottoming: How can you relax rectal muscles you don't have conscious control over? Or to put it more simply, how can you train a muscle to relax if it won't listen to you? In a way, Sexhalation is a kind of biofeedback system. But don't worry, we're not going to wheel out an electronic console and stick a Geiger counter up your ass. You can meet your biofeedback device by simply wiggling your finger. Yes, we're going on a road trip into the wilds of your rectum and I'm going to be the back seat driver.

It's best to do The Sexhalation Method after you shower when you're squeaky clean. You should know that most people will not have a close encounter of the brown kind when they explore themselves anally because the anal canal and rectum are not storage containers for feces. They are passageways for the feces to move from the sigmoid colon out to your sphincter. It is a myth that your rectum stores feces. The only time feces enter the rectum is when pressure sensors notify the brain of the need to defecate. The feces then move from the sigmoid colon in mass through the rectum and out the anal opening. Depending on your diet and fiber intake, the feces should move through the rectum and anal canal leaving little if any residue.

As we go through the Sexhalation exercises I want you to keep something in mind: Practice gives you skills. Skills give you competence. And competence gives you confidence. By the time you are done with these exercises you will approach bottoming with so much confidence (and so little anxiety) that you will practically guarantee yourself a pleasurable experience. Now, get yourself comfortable, make sure you're alone, and haul out the lube because you're about to experience…

The Sexhalation Method.

Step 1: Put lube on your finger and your anal opening.

It doesn't matter what kind of lube or which finger you use. Like the kind of guy you're attracted to, it's strictly a matter of personal preference.

Step 2: Gently press your finger against the anal opening.

Do not insert. Just keep your finger pressed gently but firmly on the opening to your anus. Stay here for a few moments and let your finger feel what's happening to the external sphincter. Notice what thoughts you have. Make sure, however, that you're pressing on, not just touching, the sphincter. Again, press but don't insert.

Step 3: Take Three Practice Pattern Breaths.

Get your body in sync with pattern breathing. Inhale deeply (through your nose only) to a slow count of four. Keep the inhalation steady. In other words, don't use up three quarters of your inhale by the time you reach a count of two. Keep the inhalation at a steady pace. At the end of the inhalation pause for a full second. Then exhale (through your nose) for a count of six. Why six seconds and not four? Studies show this is the optimal breath pattern for muscle relaxation. Again, pace yourself so the exhale is steady throughout the six seconds. At the end of the exhale, pause for a full second, then repeat the cycle.

Do this three times. Right before the fourth inhale, bring your attention to your finger, which is gently, but firmly pressed against your anal opening. Then...

Step 4: Inhale to a count of four while tightening your sphincter as hard as you can.

Keep your finger gently pressed, but not inserting into, your anus. Keep a steady count to four until you get to the end of the inhale. Pause for a second and...

Step 5: Relax your sphincter as you exhale.

Remember to exhale to a count of six. You are not pushing your finger in during the exhale—*your sphincter is relaxing onto the finger*, which is gently but firmly placed against it. Only draw in as far as the exhale/relaxation allows. If you feel discomfort or pain, you've just violated your No Pain Contract, so back off. Remember, you should <u>never</u> feel pain. Pain is a signal you're doing it wrong—you're either pressing too hard or going in too fast.

How much of your finger got drawn in? An inch? One eighth of an inch? It doesn't matter. What matters is that you just experienced the secret to pain-free bottoming:

You don't insert a penis into your rectum; you relax onto it.

This is an important concept to understand and apply. Inserting an object into the anal canal guarantees a tightening of the sphincter muscles. But relaxing onto it guarantees a loosening of them. Do this: Palm down, clench your left fist tight, tight, tight. Now try to force the index finger of your right hand into your clenched fist. Make it a battle. Notice the clenched fist will win. Now, press the index finger gently but firmly against the clenched fist without trying to force it in. Inhale to a count of four as you clench the fist as tight as you can. Now, loosen the clenched fist as you exhale to a count of six. Notice how a bit of your finger went in without actually having to forcefully insert it? This concept works with your fist and it works with your sphincter muscles. Again:

Don't insert something into your butt;
allow your butt to draw it in.

Sexhalation is combination of pattern breathing, progressive muscle relaxation and systematic desensitization. It's so effective because it is working with anatomy, not against it. A relaxed sphincter releases *downward*. When it tightens, it contracts *upward*, drawing in whatever it was relaxed onto. This release downward/contract upward process facilitates an interesting anatomical phenomenon: A small vacuum that literally sucks a part of the finger in.

To fully experience the small vacuum created by Sexhalation, try doing Steps 1-5 while you squat all the way down to the floor, balancing on the balls of your feet, with your knees forming a "V." Notice that a lot more of your finger gets drawn in and on a quicker pace. But what I really want you to feel is the suction that gets created when your sphincters relax.

Sexhalation is so key to pain-free bottoming that it's worth explaining again: You inhale as you press your finger onto *but not into* your consciously clinched sphincter. Then you exhale to relax the sphincter onto your finger. Whether you do it with a finger, a sex toy or finally, a penis (yay!) it's critical to establish a psychological and physical rhythm to insertion. Your body will start to understand (and react favor-ably) to the rhythm—inhale to tighten, exhale to loosen. Inhale to tighten, exhale to loosen. Once again:

> *You are not inserting your finger;*
> *you are drawing it in.*

In fact, I want you to use The Sexhalation Method when you do your Kegel exercises: Clench your sphincter as you inhale to a count of four. Relax the sphincter as you ex-hale to a count of six. Do this ten times a day. It will pay dividends in an unexpected place: The toilet. Learning to relax your sphincter by pairing pattern breathing with progressive muscle relaxation will ensure smooth, effortless bowel movements that will prevent hemorrhoids and fissures that come from straining too hard.

Now that you have your finger up your ass, let's move on.

Step 6: Let Your Sphincter Get Used To The Presence Of Your Finger.

Once you draw your finger in (no matter how little), keep it there without moving. As your anus realizes it's not under attack you will feel the sphincter muscles relaxing further. If you really pay attention you'll feel both sphincters. They feel like two sep-arate rings with about a quarter of an inch of flesh between them. Squeeze and relax your anus. Notice that the external sphincter relaxes on command while the internal sphincter does not. You can actually feel it tightening and relaxing spontaneously in pulses, as if it had a mind of its own. Don't do anything, just notice it.

Keep your finger in there long enough and you'll physically feel the internal sphincter—the one that does not obey conscious commands— relax around your finger. Feel it? You just experienced a great lesson: If you're patient enough the muscles you can't consciously control will unconsciously release. It's a simple law of physics. Do this: Clench your fist as hard as you can. Keep it tightly clenched as long as you can. You'll notice that after a period of time the muscle simply gives out. It cannot sustain the same level of tension forever. This brings us to another key concept in pain-free bottoming:

> *Your internal sphincter will relax*
> *if you let it let go.*

This requires patience, of course. But you saw "first hand" how the internal sphincter released on its own if you stayed still long enough. Okay, let's keep going. At this point your sphincter muscles should be so used to the inserted finger that you liter-ally can't feel much of anything. Now you're ready to continue the Sexhalations...

Step 7: Inhale as you clench your sphincter around your finger.

Remember, to a count of four—through your nose at a steady pace. Keep your finger pressing (but not inserting further) against the clenched sphincter muscles. As you reach the end of the inhale, pause for a second, then...

Step 8: Exhale as you release the sphincter muscles, allowing them to draw in more of your finger.

Notice that a tiny bit more of your finger got drawn in. Remember, you signed a no-pain contract. If you feel pain, BACK OFF or I'm going to slap a breach of contract suit on you.

Step 9: Lather. Rinse. Repeat.

Repeat steps 1-8 until your sphincter muscles have drawn in your entire finger or you simply want to stop because you don't want to miss the next episode of Family Guy. Stop whenever you feel like it. Why? Because you said so, that's why. You are in control over every aspect of bottoming and your practice sessions are no exception. Besides, it's better to quit and think you could have gone further than to continue and think you went too far. This is not a sprint; it's a marathon.

Practice, Practice, Practice.

You should repeat The Sexhalation Method as often as you can (daily is best). Do it for just a few minutes. Do it in different places (bedroom, shower) and different posi-tions (on your back, on your side, on all fours, squatting). You'll notice that your fin-ger goes in comfortably a little bit further every day. This is because each day you're stretching the sphincter muscles just a smidge, and like any muscle that gets stretched, it becomes more flexible, supple and relaxed. Try moving your finger in a circular motion while it's in there. Experiment with in and out and back and forth motions. There is no right or wrong, only what you like or don't like. Find out.

Once you can get your finger in completely without any discomfort whatsoever, experiment by gently pressing on different points of the anal canal. Did I mention *gently*? Remember, a quarter of an inch feels like a foot and half in your ass.

It's Time For Sex...With Yourself.

Masturbate and orgasm with your finger inside. Pay particular attention to what happens to your sphincter muscles as you ejaculate, indeed the entire puborectal region. Notice how all the muscles and tissue contract rhythmically. Visualize this happening around a penis inside you, how your southern region will massage it during orgasm, delivering a delicious sensation to your partner. Remember, imagery is an important aspect to Sexhalation. You're not doing this to fill your orifice; you're doing it to experience a psychological, emotional, physical and sexual high. You are submitting to a hard cock—enjoy the anticipation and heighten it with imagery that's meaningful to you. What does the penis you're submitting to look like? How is it shaped? How big is it? How thick is it? What about the guy topping you? What does he look like, smell like, feel like? What does he say to you? Is he kind and loving? Aggressive and demanding? Does he make you feel loved or demeaned? Details matter in sexual imagery. Fire up your imagination. The stronger the imagery the more enjoyable your Sexhalation exercises will be.

How To Find Out What Bottoming Will Feel Like Without Actually Doing It.

A great deal of the pleasure you get from bottoming comes from the penis stimulating the prostate as it thrusts in and out of the rectum. You can get a "sneak preview" of what that will feel like by massaging your own prostate as you masturbate.

Before I show you how, let's talk a little more about the prostate, which many people call, "The male G-Spot." The prostate is a walnut-sized gland located between the bladder and the penis (just in front of the rectum). It produces fluid that nourishes and protects sperm. During orgasm it squeezes this fluid into the urethra where it mixes with sperm and comes out as that whitish semen many of us think of as the nectar of the Gods. In fact, the prostate produces almost all of your semen.

Obviously, the prostate is crucial to your experience of orgasm. You know that moment of "ejaculatory inevitability" when you're about to come and you feel it deep inside you before anything comes out? That's because orgasm starts with the contractions of the internal sex organs (vas deferens, seminal vesicles and the prostate). Therefore, stimulating the prostate in just the right way can create enormous sexual excitement. In some men, simply stroking the prostate can make them spontaneously orgasm. But the truth is, prostate stimulation is not a universal pleasure and it accounts for a great deal of the reason that some men don't like bottoming even when it's pain-free.

Use a modified version of The Sexhalation Method to massage your own prostate:

Step 1: Gently Press Your Middle Finger Against Your Anus.

Lay on your back, spread your legs and press your lubed-up middle finger against the anal opening (you can use the index finger if you prefer, but the middle finger gives you more reach). *Make sure your hand is in the palm up position* (palm pointed to the ceiling). Remember, *press*, don't insert.

Step 2: Inhale To A Count Of Four And Squeeze Your Sphincter Shut.

Step 3: Exhale To A Count Of Six And Release The Sphincter.

Step 4: Repeat Until You Draw In Your Entire Finger.

Step 5: Gently Probe The Anal Wall Upwards Towards Your Navel.

The prostate is located behind the anal wall in the direction of your belly button (two to four inches from the sphincter). Be careful! The prostate is very sensitive. Do not poke and prod. Caress and stroke. Press gently. Use feather-light touches. You're looking for a walnut-sized fleshy ball hiding behind the anal wall. Finding it is a little like playing hide-and-seek, only you're using your finger rather than your eyes.

Step 6: Find And Trace The Contours Of The Prostate.

Once you locate it, trace your finger around the gland. Take a tour. Notice where it is. Make a mental note of how far in (and up) you had to go so that you can use this memory as a GPS for the next hide-and-seek adventure. Ask yourself how stroking your prostate feels. Good, bad? Pleasurable? Ambivalent? Don't judge; notice.

> *Can't find your prostate or not sure if you have?*
>
> The easiest way to find your prostate is to make sure you're sexually aroused. Your penis isn't the only thing that gets full and erect when you get excited—so does the prostate. So much so that it bulges into the anal wall, making it very easy to find. During arousal the prostate fills with semen fluid. The closer you get to orgasm the firmer the prostate becomes and the easier it is to find and stroke.
>
> You can also try different positions. For example, some guys have better luck laying on their left side and putting their right hand behind their back while bending the knee of the top leg.
>
> If you still can't find your prostate it could be that your fingers aren't long enough. The prostate lies two to four inches into your rectum (towards your

belly button). If your prostate is positioned higher than average and/or your fingers are shorter than average it can get a little tricky. Try a commercial prostate massager like Aneros or the Pro-State Prostate Massager. They're shaped to match the form of the anus.

Step 7: Massage The Prostate.

You need to exert firm pressure without pushing too hard. Firm but comfortable is your goal. Start at the top of the prostate and slowly push down toward the center. Then go back up. Then start at the bottom and slowly push upwards toward the center. Experiment with different directions to get different sensations. There's no right or wrong way to find out what you like. Be curious and try anything as long as you do it slowly, with care. The prostate actually has two lobes. If you can detect each lobe you can take turns massaging them. Don't be surprised if a couple of drops of fluid come out of your penis, even if it's not erect. This is what many doctors do to "milk" the prostate and relieve pressure in patients with enlarged prostates.

Step 8: Massage The Prostate While You Masturbate.

You may or may not have had an erection while exploring the prostate. It's now time to purposefully get one. Massage the prostate as you masturbate to climax. It is quite eye opening to feel your prostate enlarge as you're about to orgasm and then feel the entire rectum—sphincters and all—rhythmically contracting as you ejaculate.

If you want to massage your prostate during masturbation but don't want to go through the "hand yoga" contortions (let's face it, you have to go through a bit of twisting and bending to reach the prostate with your hands) try using a commercial prostate massager like the ones I mentioned above.

You can also try a more indirect route to stimulating your prostate—finding the pressure point on the perineum directly below the prostate. Do this: Put your index and middle fingers together and gently press the fingertips on the area between your anus and the scrotum. Southerners call this area, "The Tain't" because it "tain't your ass and it tain't your balls."

Start at the boundary of your sphincter and *gently* press up. Move an 1/8 of an inch toward your scrotum and press up. Keep going and you will eventually find the sweet spot—generally, it's the most sensitive spot in a most sensitive area. Try different pressures and find the touch that you like best.

Interesting tip:

You can wring the last bit of semen out of your ejaculation by doing the following: Right after you ejaculate, press your fingers upward starting at the edge of your sphincter and glide them firmly (but gently) toward the scrotum. As you reach the scrotum, clasp the base of your penis and squeeze up to the head. You are basically squeezing the last bit of toothpaste out of the tube—start at the base (the area just above your sphincter) and keep squeezing until you reach the opening (the tip of the urethra). You'll see extra semen come out that you didn't know you had in you. If you're a "dripper" after you ejaculate (you continue to drip semen even after your penis goes soft) this will completely eliminate it.

Was It Good For You?

Masturbating to climax while massaging your prostate is a good way to find out if you will enjoy bottoming without actually bottoming. Of course, it doesn't take into account the psychological pleasure of surrendering your body to another man (a HUGE part of the turn-on) but the prostate is known as the "male G-spot" for a reason and it contributes greatly to the physical sensations associated with bottoming. That's not to say you won't enjoy bottoming if prostate stimulation isn't your thing, but it's a pretty good indicator of how much you'll enjoy the physical (as opposed to the psychological) aspect of it.

Some guys find prostate stimulation unbelievably pleasurable while other guys find it extremely annoying. Some men only like it after a certain point of sexual arousal while others like it at any time. Still others don't care for it at all. Individuals vary widely. What causes ecstasy for some causes boredom in others.

It doesn't matter whether you like prostate stimulation or not. What matters is that you experience the process. It is quite astounding to feel your prostate thicken and grow inside the anal wall as you get closer to orgasm. It will give you a fascinating glimpse into your sexual response and a sense of respect for the process your body goes through to deliver pleasure. It will also give you insight as to what's happening to your partner if you're the one topping him, or hell, even if you're giving him a hand job!

Advancing Past A Finger.

Once you can draw in your entire finger *without any pain whatsoever*, it's time to go for two fingers, maybe three (stop there—don't be greedy!). Always use Sexhalations. Do not deviate. Here's why: You are training your body to automatically and unconsciously respond to the rhythm you've set. Inhale means contraction. Exhale means relaxation. With consistency and frequency, the puborectal region—including the sphincters, the sling and the rectum— will train itself to respond to the exhalation cue and relax far more deeply than it would with just conscious thought alone.

Time to play with toys. There is no substitute for a hard penis but there is a surrogate. Gentlemen, allow me to introduce you to an unappreciated and under-used object that is instrumental to pain-free bottoming: The dildo. But not just any dildo. A dildo with detailed specifications. You need to buy one that…

- Has a tapered body (the insertion point, or "head," is small and gets progressively bigger as it gets to the base).

- Is made with silicone.

- Has a flanged base (a collar at the base that prevents the dildo from getting stuck up your ass without a way of getting it out). You don't want to be the guy that has to go to the Emergency Room because his ass swallowed an object and won't burp it back out. Trust me, there's nothing fabulous about a trip to the ER. The lighting is bad, the outfits are ugly, and they have no concept of a VIP line.

- Is approximately five inches in length and about five inches in girth at its thickest point. Why? Because those are the dimensions of the average erect penis.

We are going to use The Sexhalation Method on the dildo but before we get to that, let's talk about something you're probably stuck on—that last statement I made about the size of the dildo you should buy. The average penis is 5" x 5"? How can that be?

There are two widely recognized ways of measuring a penis. The first is the "You Wish" method first popularized by gay dating and hookup sites. It involves looking at your pinky and seeing a thigh.

I'll talk about the second, more accurate way in a minute. First, the bad news: the average penis size is not six inches. The "six inch myth" got started when Kinsey did his landmark penis size study back in the 50's. Although there were 2,000 men in his study, it had a fatal flaw—the results were self-reported. Men were asked to go into a room, get themselves hard and measure themselves. Now tell me, would you believe anything a man says while he's holding his dick?

Men lie about size. Why do you think we came up with maps that associate an inch with a mile? Realizing that too many men were backdating their stock options, urologists developed a new way of measuring the size of the prize: A third party. So, now every legitimate penis study includes medical staff either doing the measuring or supervising it.

The most reliable study of penis size to date appears to be out of the University of California, San Francisco (where else?). Researchers let 80 men measure themselves with an observer present (don't ask, I'm just reporting it). And guess what? The average erect penis size dropped a <u>whole inch</u> from Kinsey's study, to 5.1 inches! In other words, left to their own devices, men lie. Shocking isn't it?

Here are the stats from the groundbreaking study:

- Average Length: 5.1 inches.

- Average erect girth: 4.8 inches.

- Average flaccid length: 3.5 inches.

- Average flaccid girth: 3.8 inches.

If you want to know your exact measurements, here's how to do it:

1. **Get undressed in a warm room**. "Shrinkage" will occur if it's cold. I don't know about you, but I want every millimeter counted.

2. **Use a cloth ruler.** Tape measures or straightedge rulers don't measure curvatures well.

3. **Lie on your back and start where the base of your penis meets your stomach.** In other words, measure the side of your penis facing your stomach, not the ceiling. Do NOT start from the back of your balls. Nobody includes the basement when they quote the height of a skyscraper, so don't include the tip of your ass in quoting yours.

4. **Round up to the nearest centimeter.** Not the nearest foot.

5. **Read it and weep.** Most men will fall between four and six inches, with the average being 5.1 inches.

Actually, there's a much faster and easier way to measure your cock. You don't even need to get hard to do it. All you have to do is stretch your flaccid flogger and measure it from the penopubic region to the tip. Believe it or not, every major study shows a high correlation between erectile and flaccid/stretched length.

When all is said and done, the majority of us will fall somewhere near 5.1 inches in length and 4.8 inches in girth. Skip the weepy letters about how awful it is to have an average-sized dick. Studies show there is no, as in none, as in nunca, proof that having a big dick leads to greater sexual satisfaction.

> *Interesting Tip To Share At Your Next Cocktail Party:*
>
> If you want to find out if you have a big dick without measuring it, then put a tube of toilet paper over your erect penis. If it slides all the way down to the base, you're average or below average. If it gets stuck, then pop the champagne corks because you're one of the few who have a big penis. Yes, FEW. Condom manufacturers estimate that only 6% of the population needs extra-large rubbers.

Back To The Sexhalation Method.

Okay, sorry for the detour, let's ahem, press on. Use The Sexhalation Method on your toy until you can draw it in (notice I didn't say 'insert') all the way to the base. Here's how:

Step 1: Put lube on your toy and your anal opening.

Step 2: Gently, but firmly press the toy against your anus.

Do not insert. Just stay here for a few moments and feel what's happening to the external sphincter.

Step 3: Inhale as you clench your sphincter tightly.

Inhale deeply (through your nose only) to a slow count of four as you tighten your sphincter. Keep the inhalation at a steady pace. At the end of the inhalation pause for a full second.

Step 4: Relax your sphincter as you exhale, which will draw in the toy.

Remember to exhale to a count of six. You are not pushing the toy in during the exhale—*your sphincter is relaxing onto it.* Only go in as far as the exhale/relaxation allows. Pain is a signal you're doing it wrong—you're either pressing too hard or going in too fast.

Step 5: Let your sphincter get used to the presence of the toy.

Once it's in—no matter how far—stay still. Let your sphincters adjust. Remember, the best way of getting your internal sphincter to relax is to be patient enough to let it let go. Once you get so sensitized to the feeling it's hard to discern that anything is in there, then...

Step 6: Inhale as you clench your sphincter around the toy.

Remember, to a count of four—through your nose at a steady pace. Keep the toy pressing (but not inserting) against the clenched sphincter muscles. As you reach the end of the inhale, pause for a second, then...

Step 7: Exhale as you release the sphincter muscles, allowing them to draw in more of the toy.

Notice how much of the toy got drawn in. A lot? Great. A little? Great. See, it doesn't matter. We're looking for progress, *any* progress. Remember, if it hurts or seems like it might, BACK OFF. Pain is sign that you're going in too fast, too deep or both. When it comes to Sexhalation, there is no such thing as going too slow.

Step 8: Lather. Rinse. Repeat.

Repeat steps 1-7 until your sphincter muscles have drawn in the whole toy down to the base. Some guys will be able to do it in the first session; others will take days if not weeks. Do not judge yourself just because it's taking longer than you think it should. Your anatomy dictates the pace—some people just have a tighter puborectal region than others.

Take your time. If it takes you a month of daily, progressive, no-pain "draw-ins" (notice I didn't say 'insertions') to stretch out your sphincter so what? That's a small price to pay for a lifetime of pleasurable bottoming.

Is It Painful Or Different?

You signed a "No Pain Contract" not a "No New Sensations Contract." Sometimes it's hard to tell whether what you're feeling is discomfort or simply a new sensation that you've never experienced before. If you've never had as much as a finger up your bum, *everything* is going to feel unfamiliar, but that doesn't mean it's painful. If you're not sure ask yourself...

Is this painful or just unfamiliar?

If it's painful, back off. If it's unfamiliar, relax into it. If you truly can't tell, back off. We are in no hurry. In fact, the slower you go, the more successful you'll be.

It's Time For A Penis.

Once you can fully draw in (notice I didn't say insert) a penis-sized toy into your rectum without any pain, it's time for the real thing. Wow, you are only 5.1 inches away from getting fucked! But before we proceed to the blessed event, we need to clear something up.

Your butt.

CHAPTER SIX

How Porn Star Bottoms
Handle The Ick Factor.

Their Secrets To Getting Your Butt
Cleaner Than A Brady Bunch Rerun.

WE CANNOT HAVE A CONVERSATION about keeping yourself clean without a full understanding of a delicate subject: How you eliminate waste from your body. The fear of leaving muddy tire tracks on the sheets or your partner's penis is based on a misconception that feces are stored in the rectum. In fact, they are not. Feces are stored in the sigmoid colon, which sits above the rectum. The only time your rectum fills with stool is when the sigmoid colon fills up and needs to release it. Through a combination of anatomical structure, neural switches and reflex triggers it is impossible for stool to remain in your rectum. Now, often there is residue, for sure, and we'll talk about that later in the chapter. But for now, know that your rectum, the place that will lovingly hold and pet the penis when you're bottoming, is a pipeline, not a storage device. It is the Panama Canal between the sigmoid colon and your sphincter. Ships can only pass through; they cannot anchor.

Let's take a look at why. It'll be helpful to see a diagram of how the sigmoid colon (where the last stages of fecal matter are produced) attaches to the rectum. Click here for some enlightening diagrams: http://bit.ly/S0WM9e.

The sigmoid colon releases waste (stool) to the rectum when the body is ready for elimination and only when it is ready. There are several ways the body makes sure that things don't 'slip' into the rectum accidentally. First, the juncture between the sigmoid colon and the rectum lies at ninety degrees. The sigmoid colon is horizontal where it meets the rectum, which lies on a more vertical plane. This sharp angle stops feces from entering the rectum on their own. "Security" is reinforced by a sphincter muscle between the sigmoid and the rectum (Christ, how many sphincters do we have in our bodies!). In its natural state this sphincter is constricted and thus acts as the gatekeeper. It remains tightly shut unless it receives a command from headquarters.

As fecal content grows in the sigmoid colon it exerts pressure on this sphincter muscle. This triggers one of many involuntary "defecation reflexes" and signals the sigmoid sphincter to open up and let the fecal content into the rectum. The entry of feces into the rectum distends the rectal wall. There, stretch receptors trigger signals to the descending and sigmoid colon to increase peristalsis (the involuntary constric- tion and relaxation of the muscles, creating wavelike movements that push the fecal contents forward). These "waves" of movement pass through all the way to the anus, causing the puborectal sling to loosen, straightening the S curve in your rectum, and causing the internal sphincter (remember him, the one who doesn't obey your orders to relax?) to completely relax (the bastard!).

But defecation only happens once you release the external sphincter, which you have conscious control of. When you can't find a bathroom (and you'd rather not relieve yourself on the carpet) you can clench your external sphincter to keep it from hap- pening. You will also be aided by the sling, which acts as "continence muscle" that stops you from farting or taking a shit in the middle of a cocktail party. When you need to go but can't, the sling responds to the pressure by contracting, which holds the feces back until you have the opportunity to find a bathroom.

Nice, huh?

Interesting Aside:

If you're able to prevent defecation long enough by consciously clenching your external sphincter, the stool in the rectum is often returned to the colon by reverse peristalsis, temporarily reducing pressure in the rectum (deactivating the stretch receptors). The stool is then stored in the sigmoid colon until the transverse and descending colon, which connects to the sigmoid from above, triggers the next peristalsis movement. You only want to delay defecation in cases when there are no bathrooms or you're stuck in some circumstance that prevents you from accessing one (accepting an Oscar for Best Supporting Bottom, for example). If defecation is delayed long enough, the fecal matter may harden and oh, dear, you'll get as constipated as Ru Paul when he's out of drag.

So what does all this have to do with bottoming? A lot. First, understanding the process of elimination helps reassure you that the rectum does not store feces. This should put you at ease: You will not release a shit bomb if you bottom.

Second, there are parallels between elimination and insertion. If you want objects to make a smooth entrance, it behooves you to understand how they make a graceful exit. For example, let's take that sling inside you. It pulls the lower rectum forward toward the belly button up to 90 degrees (see diagram: http://bit.ly/T3FhJj), creating an S curve. The tighter the sling, the more pronounced the S curve. The sling prevents things from leaving the rectum (it's one of the reasons you strain in the toilet) and prevents things from entering it (it blocks the penis by greeting it with the rectal wall). So let's study how the sling releases for elimination because we can use that knowledge to release it during insertion.

During defecation the sling loosens so much it decreases the S curve from almost ninety degrees to 15 degrees (almost straight) causing the external sphincter to relax involuntarily. If you can master that loosening of the sling during sex, bottoming will be a breeze. While you cannot consciously relax the puborectal sling, there are positions that naturally straighten it. Positions like the ones you take when you go to the bathroom.

Normally, you sit on the toilet with hips and knees at about a right angle. It's known as the "Catcher's position" because it's so close to the position baseball catchers take during a game. But since toilets were only invented in the nineteenth century, a good part of the world doesn't use the "catcher's position" for elimination. They use a "squatting toilet" (fancy for a hole in the ground). This forces you to squat all the way down to your ankles.

Many proctologists believe that the catcher's position we use in the western world creates bowel movement problems because it does not sufficiently loosen the puborectal sling. This keeps the S curve fairly pronounced, causing many people to strain in the bathroom. In fact research shows people strain three times greater in a sitting position than a squatting one.

Whoa, whoa! Enough of this shit! What does all this discussion about defecation postures have to do with bottoming? Again, the S curve that makes it harder for things to go out your butt is the same S curve that makes things hard for things to go in it. The "catcher's position" you take on the toilet is most like the missionary position in bed— on your back with knees raised at ninety degrees to your torso. That straightens the S sling a bit but not by a lot. But the squatting position significantly straightens out the S curve. And that is why you should start bottoming by squatting on top of your partner rather taking the missionary position. You will be shocked at how much easier a penis goes in this way. Why? Because squatting releases the sling, which straightens the S curve.

This also brings us to another point worth mentioning. Many guys feel like they have to defecate when a penis enters their rectum. Why is that? If you review the early part of this chapter you'll remember that the rectum has "stretch sensors." When the rectum is full, stretch receptors fire, giving you the feeling that you have to take a dump. When a penis enters the rectum, it sets off these stretch sensors, in the way your cat might set off the fire alarm. In other words, that feeling that you have to take a dump? It's a false alarm. This sensation will wane as your rectum learns to re-interpret the presence of a penis. It is not possible for you to have a bowel movement during sex, even if it feels like you need to.

The Best Way To Get Yourself Clean.

Although the anal canal and rectum are not storage devices for feces, it's not exactly like you can eat off your anus like it were Aunt Edna's kitchen floor. In our Sexhalation exercises you'll note that when you pull your finger out, it's mostly clean but it won't win the starring role in a Purell commercial. Like a good courtroom lawyer, you will always find evidence that a grime was committed. And if you do some finger excavating to root out the brown evil you will note that while there is no fudge, there might be sludge and even the occasional brown booger. How can you get yourself clean? Like most problems, the best way to solve this one is to avoid it in the first place. Even porn star bottoms (whether they use drugs or not) know the only way to do that is to...

Improve Your Diet.

Does your underwear look like Jackson Pollock aimed his ass at the canvas and yelled, "FIRE!"? Does your rectum look like it hosted a NASCAR event? If you do a little finger mopping up there and come out with more than just a faint residue (there will always be a little) you can bet the culprit is your diet. Specifically, you are not eating enough fiber or drinking enough water. Fiber is responsible for:

- **Keeping your shit together.**

  Soluble fiber (like bananas) dissolves in water but isn't digested, so it absorbs excess liquid in the colon, forms a thick gel and adds lots of bulk to your feces as it parades up Intestinal Hill and down to Rectum Road. Like most gay pride parades, it picks up hitchhiking stragglers. It also softens and pushes through impacted fecal matter. The fiber, I mean, not gay pride. Though you could make a case for that, too.

- **Shaping your shit.**

  Ever see those old videos of Tokyo transit police pushing passengers in with those sort of giant Schwab sticks so they can squeeze more people into the train? That's what insoluble fiber (like broccoli) does. Since it won't dissolve in water and can't be absorbed by the body, it passes through your stomach essentially intact, compacting brown "passengers" into the intestinal train and giving them the best shape to go through the colon and out your anus without breaking off and leaving unwanted specimens.

Fiber Is Your Ticket To Cleanliness.

By "bulking up" waste matter and shaping it for easier transit, fiber ensures that feces leave the rectum and anal canal virtually intact, leaving you with just a smidge of sludge, a slight residue that's easy to clean with just a little finger mopping. The problem is that you most likely suffer from a serious fiber deficiency. How do I know? Because the American Dietetic Association says so. Take a look at their stats:

Recommended Fiber Intake For Men:	30-38 grams*
Average Fiber Intake For Men:	10-15 grams

*Some experts believe it should be as high as 60 grams.

Think about this—the average guy eats less than half the recommended amount of fiber! And then they wonder why their rectum looks like a landfill? You've learned how to bottom without pain; now it's time to do it without stains, and the only way you're going to do that is to add a lot more fiber to your diet. Remember, there is no clean rectum without fiber adding bulk to the waste in your colorectal system and shaping it for easy transit out of your anus. Your mission, should you decide to accept a clean rectum, is to consistently eat about 40 grams of fiber a day. Here are a few tips on how to do that through diet alone:

1. Eat foods that are high in soluble fiber.

Soluble fiber dissolves easily in water, forming a gel-like substance that absorbs water and makes the bowel contents stickier, which binds more waste to it. This slows the speed that foods move through the stomach, making you feel fuller longer and helping you maintain or lose weight. The slow transit time is incredibly helpful if you suffer from diarrhea. Soluble fiber also softens your stool so it can pass through your system more comfortably. It also lowers the levels of LDL cholesterol and improves your ability to control your body's blood glucose level. What's not to like? Examples of soluble fiber: bananas, apples, brown rice, white beans.

2. Eat foods that are high in insoluble fiber.

Insoluble fiber doesn't dissolve in water. In fact, it passes through your intestines intact and that's why it increases stool bulk. It's also why it accelerates transit time, relieving constipation. Examples of insoluble fiber: Kale, lentils, pears.

Now, if you're reading this carefully you'll note the following:

- Soluble fiber slows transit time, relieving diarrhea.

- Insoluble fiber speeds transit time, relieving constipation.

How can this be? Will fiber confuse your body, making your rectum shit or go blind? No, soluble and insoluble fiber are the answer to both diarrhea and constipation because they regulate digestion for smooth bowel movements, which is critical to keeping you clean for bottoming.

Most fiber-rich foods contain both soluble and insoluble fiber, yet most food labels — and health sites—don't make a distinction between the two and simply list the overall fiber content of a food. How can you find out which foods have the highest soluble and/or insoluble fiber? By clicking on this terrific chart by commonsensehealth.com. It's by far the most useful fiber chart I've ever seen. Use it to balance the two types of fiber in your diet. You can also calculate the fiber in your meals by using WebMD's dietary fiber calculator. Click here: http://www.webmd.com/diet/healthtool-fiber-meter.

Porn Star Bottoms All Say That What They Eat Affects Their Ability To Bottom.

There is remarkable agreement among those in the porn industry that what you eat—and when—has a dramatic effect on the clean factor. Here's what a famous (or rather, infamous) porn star bottom told us:

> *"1 to 2 days prior to the shoot date, you want to eat as light as possible. Breakfast for me would have been an egg hard-boiled, and lunch grilled chicken, and a side salad, and I would probably do the same thing for dinner. So the majority of that diet is lean meats and fibers, no carbohydrates. I drink water and teas, and stay away from carbonated sodas because they would also – the last thing you want to do before a scene is eat or drink anything that would make you gassy."*

What If Diet Alone Can't Get You To Your Fiber Goals?

It's much better to get fiber through your diet, but this being Fast Food Nation, it won't hurt for you to take fiber supplements. The main drawback to supplements is that they lack the vitamins, minerals, and antioxidants you get from eating high fiber foods like fruits, whole grains, and beans.

The kind of fiber supplement (psyllium, methylcellulose, wheat dextrin) or brand (Konsyl, Metamucil, Citrucel, etc.) you take or the forms you take it (pills, powder, caplets, gummy bears) don't really matter. They all behave in pretty much the same way. The most common source for fiber supplements is psyllium, which comes from the seeds of a plant species called Plantago Ovata. When the husk of these seeds is placed in water they expand in size and take on a gel-like consistency. This gel-like mass soaks up water and adds bulk to your stool.

In powder form these supplements taste like sawdust sprinkled with sweeteners. Fortunately, many come in pills and capsules, which is good because I know how much you like to swallow. I kid. Start with the minimum dosage in the bottle and work yourself up. S-L-O-W-L-Y. Too much fiber at one time can make you bloat, pass gas and create unenviable digestive issues. Remember, bedrooms are No Fart Zones. You don't want your partners dying of auto-not-so-erotic asphyxiation. A couple of things you should know about taking fiber supplements:

- Spread your fiber intake throughout the day. Don't take the full dose only at night. Spread it evenly throughout the morning, afternoon and bedtime.

- Take medications at least one hour before fiber supplements or two hours after. Fiber is known to absorb certain medicines, diverting them from your body.

- Drink lots of water. Did I say a lot? Because I meant A LOT. Taking fiber without water is like bottoming without lube. It's going to hurt like hell. Drink at least eight ounces of water with every dosage.

What If You Have Stomach Problems?

A lot of gay men have IBS (Irritable Bowel Syndrome) that make their rectums a little more, ahm, messier than they like. If this seems embarrassingly true for you, I'd recommend three things:

1. **The Fiber Supplement Proven To Help IBS.**

   Calcium polycarbophil has been proven to regulate diarrhea, constipation, bloating and abdominal pain in patients suffering with IBS. Choose from the following brands and work up slowly from one gram a day to six: Fibercon, Konsyl, Fiber-tab, Fiber-Lax or Equalactin.

Even if you don't have IBS you might consider using calcium polycarbophil, a synthetic form of fiber rather than psyllium, which is naturally occurring. You'd think the natural stuff would be better for you but calcium poly-carbophil runs less of a risk of interacting with gut bacteria and producing unwanted gas. I guess it's the drag queen equivalent of fiber supplements—more real in its fakeness than even the genuine stuff.

2. A Prebiotic.

A prebiotic is essentially food for probiotics (the "good bacteria" in your gut), which promote digestive health. The one that has the most science behind it is Inulin. Because it's not digested or absorbed in the stomach it settles in the bowels where the "good" bacteria (probiotics) feed on it, thus improving bowel function (inulin is a natural compound found in a wide variety of fruits, vegetables and herbs). Brands with inulin include Metamucil Clear & Natural, Fiber-Choice, and Benefiber. Take as directed. Inulin stays in your gut and helps the "good" intestinal bacteria grow. You might want to consider taking psyllium along with inulin. Some studies show great promise in using both substances to help treat IBS.

3. A probiotic

Probiotics are "good" bacteria that reduce the growth of harmful bacteria and promote a healthy digestive system. Is that vague enough for you? While it's true that probiotics are recognized as beneficial to the digestive system, there are 400 types of probiotic bacteria in your gut. The best known of the probiotics is Lactobacillus acidophilus, which is found in yogurt with live cultures. It is not known which probiotics (alone or in combination) work to actually remedy a malady like bloating or diarrhea. There is only one probiotic that shows great promise for people with IBS or moderate-to-severe stomach problems. It's called Bifidobacterium infantis 35624. Several well-respected studies like this one (http://www. ncbi.nlm.nih.gov/pubmed/15765388) from the National Center Of Biotechnology Information show that it significantly reduces abdominal pain/ discomfort, bloating/distention, and bowel movement difficulty.

There is only one brand that sells Bifidobacterium infantis 35624. It's called Align, and it's sold pretty much at drug stores everywhere. Unfortunately, it's the costliest probiotic out there. Fortunately, it's also the most effective one, if you ask me. Within four weeks I experienced a noticeable, significant reduction in stomach problems.

How To Tell How Dirty Your Rectum Is Without Inserting A Finger.

Look down. Not at your underwear; the toilet. The size, shape and color of your poo will determine how much residue is left in your rectum. Let's start with the sound your stools make as they hit the toilet water. I'd like to quote Dr. Mehmet Oz's unfor-gettable observation:

> *"You want to hear what the stool, the poop, sounds like when it hits the water. If it sounds like a bombardier, you know, 'plop, plop, plop,' that's not right because it means you're constipated. It means the food is too hard by the time it comes out. It should hit the water like a diver from Acapulco hits the water [swoosh]."*

After hearing the swoosh sound (hopefully) look down. Your stool should be an S shape. That signifies that the stool is firm enough that it doesn't break off in little pieces, but soft enough so it doesn't hurt coming out.

Don't worry about the frequency of your bowel movement. It can be as often as three times a day or as infrequent as three times per week. There is no normal; only what's normal for you. You're better off paying attention to what the bowel movement smells like than anything else. Healthy bowel movements should not force the next person using the bathroom to wear a biohazard suit. Strong or foul-smelling stool means there's something wrong with what you're eating.

The Fibrous Conclusion.

Eating enough fiber is the only way to make sure that you can bottom without stains or odors. Fiber improves the passage of feces through your colon so that it comes out soft but firm, sweeping up stragglers and leaving no remnants in the rectum as it exits your anus. Fiber is not going to make the boys at Brita raise a glass of your butt spit and say, "Now THAT'S filtered water!" But it will ensure that you'll never have an ugly "shit bomb" episode that scars you—and your lacy white curtains—for life.

CHAPTER SEVEN

A Device That's Better Than
A Douche Or An Enema.

Enemas and douches are a bad idea.
Here's a better one.

LET'S REVIEW. THE RECTUM does not store feces. The sigmoid colon does. The rectum is the tunnel, the Panama Canal, if you will, between the sigmoid colon that stores feces and the anus, where it empties out of. While eating enough fiber guarantees safe passage without any nuggets snagging in the rectum, there will always be some residue. If fiber takes out 95% of the worry, there's still that 5% that might make you think twice. Most people think that the only way to clean out those last few percentage points is to…

Go Behind Enema Lines.

But they're wrong. Medical experts agree: Enemas are harmful. Pushing water or a mixture of water and chemicals up your bum creates a powerful peristalsis (accom-panied by bloating and cramping) that "evacuates" everything in your lower intestin-al tract. Medically, enemas are most commonly used to bring on bowel evacuation as a way of cleaning you out for a colonoscopy (an examination of the bowels with a fiber-optic camera). You can buy these kinds of enemas at drug stores (Fleet is the most popular brand. I love the name. It's like the manufacturer bought a fleet of vehicles that drive the stool through the Holland Tunnel).

Do enemas work? Yes, you'll never be cleaner in there (or up there, as the case may be). Should you do it? Absolutely not. Never, ever put chemicals up your butt without medical supervision. Even "harmless" chemicals like mild hand soap, baking soda or sodium phosphate can irritate the colon, cause cramping, and draw electrolytes from the body. But these dangers are entirely beside the point. If your rectum is so dirty that you have to hose it out, the answer isn't a fire hydrant connection; it's a better diet. Go back to the last chapter and put yourself on a fiber plan. It won't just help you bottom without stains; it'll help in a lot of aspects of your health.

But What About Plain Water Douches?

Stay away from them. Douching could have some serious negative effects. First, fre-quent douching (even if it's just plain water) may compromise the natural protective fluids and lining in your anus. An intact mucus layer protects your rectal tissues from abrasions, tears or cuts that could endanger your health. Studies show that frequent douching compromises the rectal mucosa leading to increased risk of transmission of HIV and hepatitis. There are actually two ways you can compromise the health of anal tissues—first by water removing some or all of the mucus layers and second, by poking yourself too hard with the insertion point of the douching device, which can cause microscopic tears.

Further, overuse of douching can seriously inhibit normal bowel movement. Water in the intestinal tract creates a downward peristalsis to evacuate it. Your body can lose its ability to create a natural peristalsis to evacuate your bowels, resulting in "douche dependency" to have a bowel movement. Meaning, you won't be able to take a dump without douching first.

Perhaps the grossest aspect of douching is what's called "residual liquid." You know this term as "Anal leakage." Yes, anal leakage will occur, often hours after you've fin-ished douching. Let me state the obvious: Gravy is only good on mashed potatoes. If you absolutely insist on douching then do it rarely. Limit it to special events—your first time bottoming or some other special occasion that requires a porn-quality sphincter.

Using douches or enemas aren't just unhealthy—they're impractical. You have to wait two or three hours after your last meal and at least two hours before sex to avoid latent anal leakage. Now that I've told you it's a bad idea to douche on a regular basis, it stands to reason that…

Porn Star Bottoms Douche All The Time.

Are you getting the sense that following porn star regimens is dangerous to your health? Now, why would they do something that's so detrimental to themselves? Be-cause they're getting paid to entertain the viewing audience, and while regular clean-ing without douching is good enough for private sex, it isn't for public sex, where paychecks can be wiped away with the hint of a tire track.

Most porn stars go for douching's heavy-duty armaments. Forget fey Fleet enemas, they use industrial-strength, hose-to-the-faucet enema kits like the Shower Shot, which includes a diverter valve that attaches to the same pipe as your shower head, a sturdy gooseneck-type hose, and a special tubular aluminum nozzle.

It's the equivalent of pressure-washing your insides. If you're going to go this route (and I suggest you don't) heed the warning of one porn star we spoke to:

> *"I use Shower Shot and warm water. You can get it anywhere like at Walgreens, but it's like a long hose and you attach it to the shower faucet, and it shoots up. It cleans your gut that way. The first time I did it, it was painful because I didn't know you weren't supposed to turn the water full blast. And I didn't have sex for a week after that."*

Clearly, Shower Shot isn't made by Toys R Us.

Porn stars not only do the wrong thing with industrial-strength equipment, they like to do it often. One porn star told us, *"If I'm going to a shoot, I do it right before I leave the house. And then when I arrive, I do a last minute touch up."* You know, just in case there's any lining left in his anus. Another told us, *"I spend no less than one hour that morning douching if I am shooting that day. When I arrive at the scene I do a last-minute cleanup."*

Introducing The Best Way To Get Yourself Clean.

If enemas and douches pose too great a risk (and embarrassment) for frequent use, then how can you get yourself 100% clean? I'd like to introduce you to a device that will flush out fecal residue without the dangers of an enema or a douche:

The ear syringe.

Ear syringes hold about one ounce of water—enough to get the job done but far too little to remove rectal mucus or cause peristalsis and its consequent "douche depend-ency." Here's how to use it:

1. Fill the ear syringe with warm water.

2. Apply lubrication to the tip (always use a soft-tipped syringe).

3. Insert into your anus gently.

4. Squirt gently.

5. Retain for a moment. Release.

6. Repeat until the rivers run clear.

Again, the ear syringe avoids the pitfalls of normal douches and enemas: It eliminates the possibility of loosening the protective layer of mucus, won't cause "douche dependency" for bowel movements and oh, yeah, about that anal leakage thing—it removes the possibility of looking like your underwear got shot with a gravy gun. Get thee to a drug store, stat!

What if you don't have time for an ear syringe?

Sex isn't always a planned event. What if you're at the grocery store and Mr. Right Hot Now picks up a cucumber and says, "Mine's bigger." Surely you would take him up on his offer to find out. How can you make that happen without encountering a ghastly brown experience? One word: Fiber! You've been eating lots of it, right? If not, go back to the last chapter and start chewing. Fiber planning is the best way to ensure you'll be ready for anal sex at a moment's notice.

A Clean Conclusion.

Let's review. The best way to get yourself clean is to eat a high-fiber diet. It will almost completely eliminate eyebrow and nostril-raising surprises because it forms stools that leave your body intact, leaving so little residue that just a little finger mopping in the shower will do the trick. As you will, too, I'm sure.

If you're still uncomfortable with the tiny residue that might remain (you clean freak!), you can use an ear syringe with warm water to flush out your inner tiles. That leaves you virtually spotless. I now pronounce you ready to bottom without stains.

CHAPTER EIGHT

How To Bottom For The First Time.

Combining The Best Position With
The Most Pain-Free Angle Of Entry.

Missionary? Doggie-Style?
Straight in? Angled Up?
It Matters.

YOU KNOW HOW TO RELAX your internal and external sphincter because you've been practicing sexhalations every day. By now, you can "draw in" a dildo the size of the average penis all the way to the base without any pain. You're eating enough fiber to cement the government's food pyramid to the floor. This cleans you out almost completely, and for whatever residue that might remain, you flush it out with an ear syringe.

Congratulations! You're ready to bottom without pain or stains!

There's just one thing. And that's this notion you have that your partner should take charge. Most guys fantasize about bottoming with men who initiate, direct and control the encounter. They think their role is to simply respond, yield and surrender. There is nothing wrong with this notion—it's hot, actually. It's just not very realistic the first few times you experiment with bottoming. Here's why: pain-free bottoming requires you to find the best position to straighten out your S curve, estimate the best angle of entry and control the pace of Sexhalation. How are you going to do that if you relinquish control?

In addition to not knowing a single thing about the way you're built or how Sexhalation works, your partner is dealing with his own issues. Can he stay hard enough as he deals with a condom? (A must if you're not in a monogamous relationship). Can he find your anal opening in the dark? (It's harder than you think. Tip for tops: place a fingertip on it and use it as a guide). Will he feel pressured if he's saddled with total responsibility for the success of your session? Are you going to judge him if he doesn't know exactly what to do?

This is not a good dynamic for your first few bottoming sessions. You signed up for pleasure, not pain. The only way you're going to avoid pain and experience pleasure is to control the way your partner's penis goes in and out of you. And in and out. And did I mention in and out? I know that taking control might seem a bit of an irony—isn't bottoming about surrendering yourself to another man? How can you surrender when you're in control? Isn't that an oxymoron, like "jumbo shrimp" or "pretty ugly?" Not to get all Zen up on your grill, but "controlling your surrender" is one of those contradictions that defy explanation. It cannot be explained but it can be experienced, as you're about to find out.

Once you have enough experience with anal sex, you can begin to loosen the controls and be "taken" in a way that adds to the blissful experience of surrender, but for now, know this: The top is never in charge. Listen to one famous porn star top:

> *"In my personal experience it's best for the bottom to take charge. I usually penetrate them only with the head of my dick and have them hold onto my leg or hip and they would be the one to pull me more inside and a little bit more. If I'm too deep, pull me out. I work at their pace."*

For once, I can tell you unequivocally, LISTEN TO PORN STARS. If you want to experience pain-free bottoming you have to take control. And the best way to do that is to understand that...

You've Got To Do Something About That Sling.

Once you've mastered the relaxation of the internal and external sphincters (you have, haven't you?) you still have some planning to do, otherwise your partner will hit the S curve in your rectum and it will not feel good. Remember, you have a puborectal "sling" that surrounds the rectum and pulls it forward toward the navel causing it to have an S shape. Your rectum is not vertically shaped. It's shaped more like an s-hook.

This is important to know because an object entering the rectum at the wrong angle runs into the rectal wall of the first part of the S curve. And that will make you feel like a bat is beating your insides. Do this: hold your left hand up as if you're shaking hands. This is your rectal wall. Now take your right index finger and poke the middle of the palm at ninety degrees. This is the penis stabbing the rectal wall. Watch it, that hurts! Now, angle your palm (to the left) to 45 degrees and poke again. Better, but it still hurts, right? Now, raise your right finger up by a few degrees and poke. Ahh, feels nice, right? Notice the finger slides up the "rectal wall" rather than poking and jabbing at it. You are not stabbing the rectal wall because you "straightened out the S curve" (your palm) and adjusted the penis' angle of entry (your index finger).

You've just learned two important lessons about bottoming without pain: Straightening the S curve and adjusting the angle of the penis' entry will eliminate all the pain. Now, how do you adjust your S curve and what angle should you guide the penis toward? Let's investigate.

The Secret To Straightening Your S Curve.

There is only one thing that will straighten your S curve: The position of your legs in relation to your torso. The closer your legs are to your torso, the more your S curve will straighten. You're S is at its "curviest" when you're standing up or laying down with heels touching the ground. It's at its straightest when your knees are pulled up close to your chest or shoulders. Any position that creates at least a ninety-degree angle (doggie style for example) will do a lot to straighten your S curve. No position will completely straighten it, though, so you will have to make adjustments by trying different angles of entry.

The S curve varies from person to person. Some have very little curve so almost any position straightens it. Others have a curve so pronounced they have to put their feet to their ears to straighten it, and even then it won't do much. Some people's S curves have different shapes and lay in slightly different locations within the puborectal region. It's almost impossible to say which position will straighten the S curve for you —and make bottoming more pleasurable—because it's a function of your anatomy. The only way you're going to find out is to experiment. Different positions (missionary, doggie style) may or may not sufficiently straighten out your S curve, but there is *one* that will absolutely maximize it. And this brings us to…

The Best Position For Pain-Free Bottoming.

Squatting over your partner straightens out the S curve better than any single position. Millions of men try bottoming on their back, on their knees, on their stomachs and God knows what other positions, only to stop because it hurt too much. But the minute they try squatting onto an erect penis, everything changes. Why? Let's do an experiment. Get in the shower (don't take this book with you—it isn't water proof!), lube up a finger and draw in your finger (notice I didn't say insert) with Sexhalations as you stand in the shower. Notice there's a certain difficulty? Now, squat all the way to the ground and do the same thing. Notice how much easier the finger got drawn in? Amazing, isn't it? Squatting loosens the puborectal sling, allowing the rectum to straighten out so that it comes close to being vertical. The conclusion is obvious: It is far easier to draw an object into your rectum when your knees are closest to your chest. And which position draws the knees closest to your chest? Squatting.

Of course, there are some disadvantages to the squatting position. There's a certain awkwardness associated with bottoming for the first time (as there is for anything) and squatting open ups your body to visual inspection in ways that being underneath your partner does not. It can make you feel exposed and vulnerable. There is also a sense of separation from your partner because your torsos, especially the heart area, aren't touching. Some people need to feel the heat of their partner's body to feel more secure.

Still, a few moments of awkwardness is a small price to pay for being able to draw in your partner's penis easily and without pain. Squatting gives you more control than any other position. It completely avoids the clumsiness of your partner poking his penis in different parts of your butt because he can't quite find your anus (it's the gay version of playing pin the tail on the donkey). It also eliminates the possibility of him thrusting in hard and painfully, rather than you drawing the penis in with Sexhalations.

Once your partner is inside you it doesn't take much to roll over (with the penis inside you—no point in starting all over again!) to get in different positions. Of course, you don't have to start by squatting. Pick any position you feel comfortable with. This is your show and you're the star. You are not going to experience any pain if you follow all the directions.

While squatting straightens out your S curve better than any other position, it does not straighten it out completely. Although you've significantly reduced the risk, you still run the danger of your partner's penis stabbing your rectal wall. You can solve this problem by understanding...

The Best Angle Of Entry.

Remember your finger poking your left palm at ninety degrees? When you "straightened the S curve" in your palm it made it easier for the finger to move forward, although not completely. But when you raised the angle of the finger? Magic! It slid along the "rectal wall" of your palm easily and without resistance. The lesson: You—*not your partner*—must guide your partner's penis in so that it slides along the rectal wall rather than poke at it. You are the only one who can do this effectively. Only you intuitively know what path the penis should take. Only you can immediately course-correct at the hint of discomfort. Only you can do all of this at a pace that's comfortable for you. Your partner? I say this with love, but what he doesn't know about your S curve is a lot.

It's difficult to say which angle of entry is right for you because so much depends on things that are unknowable—where your S curve begins, how straightened it be-

comes in certain positions, the natural angle of your partner's penis and more. However, all things being even the best angle of entry is:

About 15 degrees *away* from your navel.

Why? Because the puborectal slings forces the first curve in your rectum *toward* the
navel, exposing more "perpendicularity" of the rectal wall to the entering penis. By
guiding the head of the penis away from the navel (but not too much!) the penis will
be more parallel to the rectal walls. This will avoid the stabbing sensation beginners
feel. Get back in the shower and do this: Squat and use Sexhalations to draw your finger in toward the navel. You'll notice how quickly you hit the rectal wall. If you keep
pressing up you'll hit the prostate (yeah, that's the sensitive jab you just felt). Imagine
what it'll feel with a penis going in that angle. Ouch! Now, pull your finger out
(slowly!) and use Sexhalations to draw in your finger, this time completely away from
the navel. Notice you didn't really feel any "stab?" That's because your finger lies parallel to the back of the rectal wall when it's fully inserted. Obviously, you don't want
the penis aiming for the back of the rectal wall (your partner would have to stretch
his penis backward). I just wanted to show you the dramatic difference between
angling the penis toward and away from the navel.

So, again, the best angle of entry is about 15 degrees away from your navel. Now,
there is something you should be aware of…

The Right Angle + A Straightened S Curve Is Not Enough To Avoid Pain.

Inserting an object into your rectum naturally tenses all the muscles surrounding the
rectum. Even a penis going in at the right angle in a straightened S curve will hurt if
the surrounding muscles tense up and clamp down. In fact, the tension and constric-
tion will tighten the sling and bring the curve back to your S with the penis still in the
rectum. Can you say "Oww!?"

Now, you can't consciously relax the S curve but you can give it the opportunity to—
by proceeding s-l-o-w-l-y. Going slow gives the muscles in the puborectal region a
chance to relax and re-interpret the insertion of the penis from "Attack!" to "Ooh,
pizza delivery!"

By the way, all anal and rectal muscles clamp down in response to fear, stress, and
anxiety—in or out of bed. When you describe an uptight guy as a "tight ass," you
aren't just commenting on his personality. Back to you: Go slow and give the rectal
muscles a chance to get acclimated so they re-interpret the presence of a penis
favorably and relax on their own. Remember what you learned about your internal

sphincter because it applies to all the involuntary muscles in the rectum: You can't force it to relax. You have to let it let go.

Once He's In, Then What?

Why are you asking me? You should be telling him. Do you need him to stay still? Tell him. Do you want him to begin thrusting? Tell him how deeply. Do you only want shallow thrusts? Ask him. Do you want to change positions? Try it. Do you want to masturbate? Then do it. My point is that you are in charge. There is no right or wrong; only what feels good and what doesn't. And while we're discussing all this, I have one last point I'd like to make:

Enjoy.

The Porn Star Secret To Successful Bottoming: Lube. If there's one thing we can look to the porn industry for medically sound insights into bottoming is its constant use of lube. Listen to what one porn director told us:

> *"Use lots of lube, way more than you probably are using now. You hear this a lot, but guys rarely actually take this advice and use enough lube. Add lube every five minutes or so. It's true that you don't see the breaks in porn videos, and those breaks are used to add lube mostly."*

Remember this and you'll never go wrong: When it comes to lube, nothing succeeds like excess.

A Penny For Your Thoughts.

So far we've only talked about the mechanics of bottoming because without them you are guaranteed to have a painful, stainful experience. But it's important to remember why you're taking this journey in the first place. This is not a science experiment and you are not a lab rat. You are bottoming for very specific, human reasons: You want to feel closer to your partner; you want to give him something of yourself. You want to feel the presence of his essence inside you. You want him to dominate you. You want to submit to him. You want to *give* him mind-numbing pleasure. You want to *get* mind-numbing pleasure from him. You've loved his cock in your hands and in your mouth and now you want it inside you. You want to feel the kind of physical, sexual union that can only come from opening yourself fully to him.

Through every step of the process—from Sexhalation to getting into a position you're comfortable with to guiding his penis in—it's important that you ignite your sexual imagination, stay present to the beauty of your partner's body and enjoy the psycho-logical and emotional journey that being penetrated offers.

The best way to infuse passion through the initial mechanics is to *simulate* bottoming before proceeding to the real thing. Get under him. Feel his heat, smell his essence, have him rub his erect penis around your anus and perineal area. Feel the heat and the hardness of his penis as he separates your legs with his thighs and grinds on you without actually penetrating you. It's a tremendous turn on. Put lube in your hand, place it behind you and have him thrust his penis into it as if it were your anus. Feel how smoothly it glides through your hand. Feel the strength and the firmness and imagine it going inside you.

Bottoming, like any sex act, is half physical, half psychological. If sex were all physical you'd lust after women, too. After all, lips are lips, orifices are orifices. But sex isn't all physical. Far from it. If you want to truly enjoy bottoming allow yourself to experi-ence what it's like to be "taken." Because you are, you know. A hard penis is penetrat-ing you. You are being "owned," however temporarily, and you should get the max-imum pleasure out of this new experience. This is erotic. It's sexy. Embrace it. Pay at-tention to the subtle and not so subtle emotions you're experiencing and remember one of my core principles about sexual fulfillment:

> *It's not what he can do to you;*
> *it's where he can take you.*

Let him take you.

A Few Conclusions To Hammer In.

Take control. Your partner has no idea how you're put together on the inside. He's likely to do everything wrong—go too fast, use too much force, and go in at the wrong angle. If you want to have a pain-free experience you have to let go of the idea that your pleasure is up to him. Laying back and letting him take charge is a guaran-tee that you will experience enormous pain. While bottoming is a submissive role, it should be a well-planned one. By taking control I mean:

- Let your partner know that you want to manage the process. He'll be grateful. Topping a newbie is actually hard work. Besides, he doesn't want to hurt you. At least not this time!

- *You* choose the position.

- *You* guide his penis in (about 15 degrees away from your navel).

- *You* decide when—and whether—you want him to start thrusting.

- *You* ask him for the kind thrusts you want him to attempt (shallow/deep, fast/slow, etc.).

Now there are just a few last tips to make the journey into your expanded sexual self a little more pleasurable:

- Try having your partner use a circular rather than a thrusting motion. Some guys initially don't like the straight in-and-out business (it can happen if you partner's penis is unusually stiff, straight or longer than average).

- Put lube on and in your anus as well as your partner's penis.

- Experiment with different positions. If missionary isn't working, for example, try resting one leg over his shoulder and the other one on the bed. Or try laying on your side, facing away from your partner as if you were spooning. Because it's a common sleeping position, it helps the body relax faster and deeper. Don't be afraid to try things that seem a little odd. If it feels good it's because your S curve straightened out and your partner's penis stimulates the prostate in a more effective way.

- Stop when it feels uncomfortable or if you need a break. This is your maiden flight. Even though following my instructions correctly will help you avoid pain, do not push yourself. Pace yourself. It's better to end knowing you could have gone longer than to end regretting that you did. Stop if it doesn't feel right, even if your partner pressures you. Sure, you might disappoint him but so what? For now, this is your show. He'll reap the benefits of patience later.

Are You Ready To Try?

Congratulations! You're ready to bottom without pain or stains! But before you try, wouldn't it be great to get a step-by-step picture of bottoming from beginning to end? It might be helpful for you to see how God's original gay couple, Adam and Steve, approached it. Let's take a look.

CHAPTER NINE

A Guided Tour Of
A Pain-Free Bottoming Session Between Adam And Steve.

A real-time, step-by-step guide that will
light you up like an all-night liquor store.

ADAM AND STEVE HAVE BEEN DATING a few months. Adam likes bottoming for Steve but he also wants to top him. They tried a couple of times but Steve was just so tight down there that they couldn't complete the act. It wasn't that Steve didn't want to bottom for Adam, it's just that the pain was so sharp he simply stopped trying. Finally they bought this book and decided to give it a try. Steve was determined not to repeat the painful experiences he had with bottoming in the past. He knew he couldn't just jump into bed and hope for the best, so he took note of the first part of this book: *Prepare*. Here's how he started:

Two Weeks Before Steve's First Attempt At Bottoming.

1. **He mentally signs his "No Pain" contract.** No pain, no way, no how, at no time. This is an enormous burden off his shoulders (and his rectum!). He can now go from someone paralyzed with "anticipatory pain" to somebody who looked forward to "anticipatory pleasure."

2. **He takes fiber supplements to make sure that his rectum stays clean.** He tried upping his fiber quotient by changing his diet, but it didn't seem to help so he decided to take supplements.

3. **He begins his "Sexercise" plan:** Kegel exercises to strengthen both his internal and external sphincter muscles.

4. **He begins doing Sexhalations with his finger.** At first, he can barely draw in 1/8 of an inch, but he doesn't get frustrated. At least the 1/8 of an inch went in without pain! He is also fascinated by the fact that he isn't *inserting* his finger as he had tried before, but "drawing it in" with a combination of systematic desensitization, pattern breathing, progressive muscle relaxation and sexual imagery. He really gets it that you don't insert an object into your rectum; *you relax onto it.* And as he gets better

and better with Sexhalations he draws in his whole finger with no pain whatsoever. Then…

A Week Before His First Attempt At Bottoming…

5. **He begins massaging his prostate when he masturbates.** Steve wants to get a good sense of his anatomy and sexual response. So he searches for, finds his prostate and massages it as he masturbates to climax. He is amazed at how much he likes it and how fascinated he is with the way his body works.

6. **He buys a dildo about the length and width of his partner's penis.** While most guys only need to buy a dildo five inches in length and five inches in girth (the aver - age size of a man's penis), Steve's partner, Adam, is bigger than average so he buys one closer to his size.

7. **He practices Sexhalations on his dildo.** He keeps to the letter of his No Pain con - tract—he progresses slowly and if he gets even a hint of pain he backs off. It's slow progress but *painless* progress. He makes a conscious distinction between pain and unfamiliarity. When he decides it's pain he backs off. When he thinks it's simply un - familiar, he stays where he is, waits for the unfamiliar to become familiar and pro - ceeds accordingly.

8. **He draws in the entire dildo without any pain whatsoever.** It takes him longer than he anticipated but Steve is amazed. He could now draw in a dildo the size of his partner's penis in his butt without any pain! He is so ready for the real thing!

9. **He buys a small ear syringe to clean himself up.** The fiber is doing its work— Steve sees a significant improvement in the cleanliness factor (there is very little evid - ence of residue in his rectum). Still, Steve is a clean freak so he buys an ear syringe. He knows he doesn't want to try it immediately before the first time he bottoms, so he does a few practice sessions a few days earlier. Steve is now ready to bottom without pain or stains! This is how his first session went.

Early Saturday Night…

10. **Steve uses the ear syringe to completely clean himself up.**

He does it earlier in the night so as not to interrupt the mood. Let's face it, there's nothing worse than interrupting a hot and heavy make-out session to stick an ear syringe up your ass.

Saturday night, midnight…

Adam and Steve make out.

They kiss deeply, undress each other and head to the bedroom.

Steve Ignites His Anticipation With Vivid Sexual Imagery.

Steve goes down on Adam, paying attention to and reveling in the size, strength and firmness of Adam's cock. He is filled with desire for it, knowing that Adam is also filled with desire for his own cock. While it's in his mouth, Steve thinks, "This beautiful cock is going to be inside me in just a few minutes. I want to be owned by it, I want to give myself up to it."

As they kiss, Adam rolls on top and covers all of Steve's body with his own—chest to chest, his hands and feet on Steve's hands and feet. Then he gently pins Steve's hands over his head and uses his knees to separate his thighs. He slides his hard dick between Steve's legs, rubbing the head of his penis softly, gently around the opening of his anus and perineum to let him feel the strength and heat of his big cock. Steve squeezes lube onto his hand, which he puts behind him, as if it were an extension of his anus. He grabs Adam's dick and Adam starts slowly, gently thrusting into his hand is if he were inside Steve. Soon, Steve is in an erotic spell. First, he had Adam's hard cock in his mouth and now he feels the heat and its strength between his legs, thrusting into his hands. Steve is ready. Adam caresses his anus with lubed fingers. Steve is going mad with anticipation. He shows Adam how to keep his finger gently pressed against his anus without inserting and does Sexhalations. In almost no time, Adam's finger is completely drawn inside of Steve, without the slightest bit of pain. Adam is shocked—he's never gone this far without Steve complaining about how much it hurts. They make out some more and Steve is rarin' to go.

Adam Puts A Condom On.

Although they're boyfriends they haven't had the commitment/monogamy discussion. Both feel, justifiably, that they should stay safe and use condoms.

Steve Straddles Adam.

As he squats over Adam's erect penis, Steve holds the head so it's angled about fifteen degrees away from his navel. He also positions himself so that this is easier to do. With the head of Steve's penis gently, but firmly against his anus, Steve begins his Sexhalations. He does not insert Adam's penis in, nor does he try to sit on it. He "draws it in" with the combination of pattern breathing, progressive muscle relaxation and systematic desensitization.

Steve Draws Adam's Penis In Very Slowly.

He purposefully goes in slow, even though he feels like he could go faster. Why? Because he knows that no matter how relaxed the sphincter, no matter how much you straighten the S curve, the puborectal muscles naturally contract when an object is inserted into the rectum. He knows he needs to let his body re-interpret the insertion from "Invasion!" to "Pizza delivery!" So he does.

Steve Makes Small Adjustments To His Position And Angle Of Entry.

He sees that even tiny changes make a big difference in the ease with which Adam's penis gets drawn in. He pays careful attention to what he's feeling and the resistance his body gives back.

Steve Notices He Doesn't Have An Erection.

Guys who bottom often don't get hard. The "sensory overload" that accompanies bottoming temporarily diverts attention away from their penis. Rather than questioning why or thinking that it's a sign that he's not turned on (it isn't), Steve just accepts it and moves on. In fact, it's probably a good idea not to stimulate yourself in the beginning, as arousal can cause the sphincters to tighten up somewhat and make penetration a little more difficult.

Steve Draws In Adam's Penis All The Way To The Base.

About a quarter of the way through, Steve notices something that amazes him. Adam's entire penis got sucked into his rectum without any effort at all. Steve wasn't drawing it in and Adam wasn't thrusting it in. It just seemed to go in on its own. This is the "vacuum effect" we talked about earlier in the book. Once it was in, Steve said, "Wow, you're completely inside me and it doesn't hurt!" Adam had a different thought: "Wow, I'm completely inside you and it feels great!"

Steve Tells Adam To Stay Still.

Steve is trying to process everything and it doesn't feel quite right for Adam to start pumping, so he says, "Stay right there. Please don't move until I get used to this feeling."

Steve Feels Like He Has To Go To The Bathroom.

He doesn't get alarmed, though. He remembers that the rectum has "stretch sensors" that activate the elimination reflex. His body senses that his rectum is full so it thinks it has to relieve itself. But there is no stool in his rectum and it's not possible for the sigmoid colon to release stool into it, and within just a few seconds, the feeling of wanting to go to the bathroom recedes, even though Steve still feels "full" (he is—he's got an eight-inch penis inside him!).

Steve Is Ready For Adam To Start Pumping.

He asks Adam to go slow. *Very slow.* As Steve gets used to the feeling—and likes it— he starts to ask Adam to go faster. But then he realizes he'd rather control the depth and speed of the thrusts, which he can do because he's on top of Adam. So he starts sitting deeper and slightly faster on Adam's cock. He decides he doesn't like Adam going in too far, so he changes the depth to his liking. Steve is constantly course cor‑ recting to eliminate the potential for pain and to maximize pleasure.

Steve Puts Adam's Hands On His Balls And Nipples.

Steve intuitively knows that he needs more stimulation so he asks for it, this time in a non-verbal way.

Steve Wants Adam To Be On Top Of Him.

He tells him and they both roll to missionary at the same time in a way that Adam's penis doesn't slip out. As Adam sees that Steve is clearly not in pain, he starts taking over. He thrusts slowly and asks Steve if he's okay, if he likes this. Steve says yes, so Adam starts pumping a bit faster and a bit deeper. Steve likes the speed but not the depth and he expresses this to Adam, who complies. Steve gets a vague feeling that he needs to urinate. This is fairly common for the receptive partner when he's on his back. That's because the bladder rests directly on the rectum. As Adam's penis pushes into Steve's rectum it prods the bladder, making Steve think he has to urinate when he doesn't. The feeling goes away once it's reinterpreted correctly.

Steve Consciously Stays Present & Activates His Sexual Imagination.

He realizes that everything so far has been about mechanics and logistics. Now that he's comfortable and all the "sensory overload" has receded somewhat, he pays atten‑ tion to exactly what he's experiencing. He loves the heat of Adam's body on top of him. He loves the very idea of Adam's big, beautiful, hard dick inside him. For the first time he feels like he's being 'taken,' like he's submitting to the strength and mas‑ culinity of a hard cock. This turns him on so much that for the first time he notices that he's getting hard.

Steve Begins To Masturbate.

This is a bit difficult because Adam is on top of him, but they both instinctively make the space for it. Steve and Adam are both lost in the feeling and amazed that they're actually having sex without pain (or stains!).

Steve Starts Feeling Discomfort.

That's because there's more pressure on and in him (there's more weight behind Adam's thrusts). Steve is not experiencing pain but it's headed there. So he asks Adam if they can try a different position. Adam says, "Let's get you on your stomach," and helps Steve get on all fours without taking his penis out.

Steve Suddenly Experiences A Pleasure He Hadn't Anticipated.

Clearly, doggie style straightened out his S curve in a dramatic way, and it probably changed the way Adam's penis stimulated his prostate. He takes note of this for the future and it isn't long before...

Steve Has His First Orgasm While Bottoming.

He's amazed at how far he shoots and how much ejaculate comes out. This isn't un-usual because the prostate is responsible for the production of ejaculate. The more stimulated the prostate gets, the more semen it will produce, and the more forcefully it will be expelled.

Steve Wants Adam To Pull Out.

Almost as soon as he ejaculates, Steve urgently wants Adam to pull out (but s-l-o-w-l-y). This is not unusual. Men typically want all sexual activity to stop after they ejac-ulate and bottoming is no different. Adam was hoping to come inside Steve but he knows what it's like to want your partner to pull out immediately so he does. Steve wants Adam to come on his chest and he does.

Steve And Adam Lay Together In Post-Coital Bliss.

They're both incredibly happy as they see new sexual horizons open up in front of them. Adam feels like he now has a fuller experience of Steve (before, Adam was always the one to bottom). Steve feels like he knows Adam in a totally different way. They feel closer to each other than they've ever been, knowing that they've traded vulnerabilities, been sensitive to each other's needs and honored each other's requests in a way that served them both.

A Few Versatile Conclusions.

Do you know why Steve's first bottoming experience was so successful? He took con-trol. Your success will depend on your willingness, like Steve, to take control and clearly communicate what you need. Only you know what you need when you need it. And if you don't, you're the only one who can find out.

The experience of bottoming is different for everyone. Some guys literally come within thirty seconds of being penetrated. Others can't get hard, even when they're enjoying it. Some guys love missionary because they like the body heat and the feeling of submission that comes from being on the bottom. Others find it suffocating and prefer less confining positions. Some guys like slow, deep thrusts, others like shallow, jackhammer thrusts. Everybody is different. *Find out what you like, not what you're supposed to like.*

A Note On Timing.

The Sexhalation Method is a powerful tool. You may be able to use it (in combination with straightening out your S curve and controlling the angle of entry) to bottom successfully without ever going through any of the training exercises (Kegels, fingers, dildo). But the reality is that most guys can't. When it comes to the ease of bottoming, anatomy is destiny. The tightness of your sphincters, the shape and elasticity of your rectum and the shape, location and severity of your S curve will determine how long it will take to train your puborectal region to accept a hard penis without any pain. Do not despair if it takes you longer than the two weeks it usually takes the average guy to do it. It doesn't mean you've failed; it means that your puborectal region is built in a way that requires more training. This isn't a race. Don't let impatience rob you of a lifetime of great bottoming experiences.

A Few Last Tips.

Use a pillow or two under your butt—it'll change the angle, ease the strain on your lower back and overall make you more comfortable.

Try to avoid doggie style at first (although Steve liked it!). This position allows the maximum insertion of the penis into the rectum, which may be uncomfortable the first few times you bottom.

Don't worry if you lose your erection or only get a partial one. While it may be a reflection of your emotional discomfort (it better not be physical discomfort—you'd be in violation of your No Pain contract!), it's just as often the case that your erotic attention shifted away from your penis to your anus. Ever notice that you sometimes experience a partial or total loss of erection when you're giving head? It's not that you're not turned on; it's that your focus is on his penis, not yours. So don't freak out if you don't get hard. Remember, everybody has different reactions.

Gas. It's going to happen. Any time air gets pushed into a small, enclosed area, it's going to create an unwanted sound at some point in the proceedings. Don't worry about it. If it happens, the only appropriate response is laughter.

Anal intercourse stimulates three areas: The prostate ("the male g-spot"), the nerve endings in the opening of the anus (the rectum itself has few nerve endings. It primarily transmits sensations of pressure.), and the "penile bulb" located at the base of the penis, just below the surface of the perineum. Guys have different reactions to having these areas stimulated. Some, like Steve, have astonishingly pleasurable reac-tions, while others have a shoulder-shrugging, is-that-all-there-is experience. Still others simply don't like any of the sensations. Where you fall in the spectrum of reac-tions is strictly a personal preference that you should not judge. Don't feel like there's something wrong with you if you didn't experience the earth move under your feet. Lots of guys try pain-free bottoming and don't like it.

Still, I'd like you to consider a core philosophy I have about sex: Never try anything once. Try it three times. The first time you'll get it wrong. The second time will be awkward, and the third time will let you experience enough of it to make a determin-ation if it's something you like.

If you were underwhelmed with your experience, don't worry about it. You've got two to go!

CHAPTER TEN

A Painless Conclusion

Bits and bobs to help you remember
the important stuff and keep you from
falling off the stupid tree and hitting
every branch on the way down.

A lawyer runs a stop sign and gets pulled over. When the cop asks for his license and registration, the lawyer asks, "What for?" "You didn't come to a complete stop at the sign," the officer says. "I slowed down, and no one was coming," the lawyer argues. "Show me the difference between 'slow down' and 'stop' and I'll accept the ticket." "Exit your vehicle, sir," the cop says. He then begins beating the lawyer with a nightstick, yelling, "Do you want me to stop or just slow down?"

IMPATIENCE IS YOUR BIGGEST ENEMY. Like the lawyer in the story you will probably get impatient, break the speed limit and end up feeling like you got attacked with a nightstick. The single most effective thing you can do to bottom painlessly is to proceed s-l-o-w-l-y. The race doesn't go to the swift; it goes to the patient.

That said, let's recap some of the highlights so I can send you off with a final note of knowledge and wisdom.

Emotional Blocks.

Don't let preconceived notions of receiving a penis between your legs stop you from having anal sex. Bottoming does not make you a woman. It does not strip you of your masculinity.

Replace your "anticipatory anxiety," or the expectation of pain, with "anticipatory pleasure" by signing a No Pain Contract. You agree to never experience pain—no way, no how, not ever. By taking the fear of pain off the table you will eliminate the "anticipatory anxiety" that stops you from bottoming or keeps you so tense you can never fully relax.

How To Overcome The Three Sources Of Pain That Stop You From Bottoming.

Kegel exercises will help tone the entire puborectal region, but especially your extern-al sphincter, which is under your conscious control. Toned muscles respond better to conscious efforts at relaxation. You can relax your *internal* sphincter, the one that's not under your conscious control, by "letting it let go" when your favorite man or man-made object is drawn in (notice I didn't say inserted). You can straighten your S-curve, a major source of pain, by experimenting with different positions. In most cases, the best position is the one that draws your knees closest to your chest. Finally, always go slow because the body automatically responds to an insertion by clenching and clamping down to expel the "invading" force. This is only an initial response, and if you go slow enough you can significantly decrease or avoid this natural tight-ening.

The Sexhalation Method.

By combining progressive muscle relaxation, pattern breathing, sexual imagery and systematic desensitization you can completely eliminate pain from bottoming. Prac-tice well and practice often. Start with your fingers and then to a toy and then to the real thing. Remember the formula: Inhale/tense; exhale/release. Inhale/tense; exhale/release. The key is consistency. *Always* use this structured breath pattern because your body will subconsciously trigger a deeper relaxation response when you are consistent with your actions. With The Sexhalation Method you'll discover some fairly profound insights about bottoming:

- Your puborectal muscles will relax more if you tighten them first.

- You will avoid pain if you concentrate on relaxing onto a penis rather than having it inserted into you.

- A relaxed sphincter releases *downward*. When it tightens, it contracts *upward*, drawing in whatever it was relaxed onto. This release downward/ contract upward process creates a small vacuum that literally sucks in the finger/toy/penis pressed against your anus.

- If you're patient enough the muscles you can't consciously control will unconsciously release. Remember to "let it let go."

Managing The Ick Factor.

The rectum does not store feces. It is the Panama Canal between the sigmoid colon and your sphincter. Ships can only pass through; they cannot anchor. Still, for some people, the rectum is a hot mess. This is a sign of fiber deficiency. You will see a dramatic improvement in the cleanliness factor if you eat a fiber-rich diet. You can speed up the process by taking fiber supplements. Do not use enemas or douches (ex-cept for special occasions) because they are harmful to your body. Instead, use an ear syringe if you don't feel that you're clean enough.

Bottoming For The First Time.

The top is never in charge. Not if you want to have a pain-free experience. Take con-trol. Your partner doesn't know how you're built on the inside, he doesn't know about The Sexhalation Method and I promise he'll go too fast, too hard, too soon. By taking control things will go your way. Remember that squatting is the best position to start with and that the best angle of entry is about 15 degrees away from your na-vel. Finally, don't forget that bottoming isn't about mechanics; it's about passion. Use vivid sexual imagery and stay present to your lover's body and energy throughout the proceedings. This is not an ordeal you're trying to get through. It's a pleasure you want to revel in.

Final Thoughts.

If you follow the instructions in this book you will be able to inhale living room fur-niture through your anus like it were a line of coke. This might make you want to bottom for the entire western world but I'd like to offer a cautionary tale against do-ing it with inappropriate people. Meet my friend, Doctor Dave. He could never bot-tom until he read this book. He wanted to try his newfound skill on multiple partners but he worked 14-hour days at his practice, so he didn't have the opportunity to meet a lot of people. Unfortunately, he ended up having sex with several of his patients. He tried to rationalize his behavior by reminding me that he was single, that his patients were single, that he wasn't the first doctor to sleep with his patients and that nobody was harmed by the experiences. Finally, he asked for my advice.

I said, "Dave, you're a vet."

My point, and I do have one, is a) never take your pets to Dr. Dave, and b) don't take sex so seriously. Let this story remind you that no matter how serious sex gets, there's always room for laughter. Thank you for allowing me to help you experience a better sex life. Now, go. Bottom. And don't forget to laugh.

CHAPTER ELEVEN

Questions About Bottoming You Never Thought To Ask.

Question:

Your advice on how to bottom without pain a while back was really good. In fact, too good. Now that I've learned how to do it without any pain, I've become a RA-GING bottom. I love the way it feels and find myself cruising for hung guys to satisfy that deep-down big-dick hunger. But I'm worried that I'm going to stretch myself out permanently and do real damage. Will I end up wearing Depends if I keep banging dudes with big dongs?

– Bottomless pit

Dear Bottomless Pitt:

Yes, if you're not careful one day you're going to bend down in your underwear and look like you've been shot with a gravy gun. Fortunately, there are ways to avoid it, but before we get to that, we need a little background. The sphincter and anal canal are remarkably elastic. During surgery, doctors can dilate the sphincter to the point of putting their hands up your ass. And no, you can't volunteer to do it without anesthesia.

Think of your butt hole as a rubber band. It springs back to its original position unless you stretch it past its ability to rebound. Nobody knows where your sphincter's rebound point is but, trust me, go past it and the only fudge you'll be packing is at the bakery.

So how do you avoid a diaper-free future? By 'training' the elasticity of your sphincter muscles. There are two ways to do it:

1. **Play With Toys.** Practice pain-free insertion with butt plugs and dildos. Insert them to the point it gets uncomfortable, back off, hold it, and when it's comfortable then push further.

2. **Play With Bigger Toys.** Assuming you don't want your butt to be so pitiful it's only worth sitting on, I'd graduate to bigger and bigger toys. But again, be careful. You know that vague burning sensation you can get when you bottom?

It's blood rushing to the area or the lining of your anus being torn. If you're used to bottoming for guys in the six- to seven-inch range and you find a ten-inch specimen, DON'T let him top you. That's what prison's for. In the outside world, DIY it with a ten-inch toy first. Remember, practice makes perfect—without perforations.

3. **Buy Lube By The Barrel**. It eases penetration and minimizes abrasions caused by skin-to-skin friction. When it comes to lube too much is never enough.

4. **Do Butt-tightening Exercises.** Exercising the pelvic floor muscles is the most important thing you can do to regain elasticity. And believe me, you don't want to regain it; you want to keep it from ever leaving. Here's a step-by-step guide on how to do them:

    ◆   *Contract and release.* Squeeze the muscles you use to stop peeing. Do ten in a row, three times a day. Then gradually increase the number of contractions.

    ◆   *Vary the exercises.* Try 'The Flutter' (tighten and let go quickly) and the 'Pinch and Hold' (tighten and don't let go till you count to fifteen).

    ◆   *Vary the positions.* Start by sitting or standing but then try it while lying on your back or side or even while squatting. Different positions tone the muscle quicker.

    ◆   *Add weight training.* Put a towel on your erect penis and do the contractions. You want bragging rights? Do them with wet towels.

Question:

My dick goes soft when a guy is fucking me. Is that normal? I enjoy being a bottom when there's chemistry between us. I like having the guy I'm attracted to inside of me, giving him the pleasure of my ass. So why do I lose my erection when it feels so good?

– Tentative Bottom

Dear Tentative:

Anal stimulation doesn't always lead to penile erections. Even in "Pizza Porn"—you know, where guys get pounded into dough and tossed up high—a lot of them don't get hard.

Surrendering yourself to another man often gives more psychic than sexual pleasure.

Of course, there's always the possibility that since you only do it with guys you really like, your body subconsciously protects you from the possibility of emotional pain by keeping you soft. It lowers the intensity of your feelings and ultimately your attach-ment to the prick that's going to run out the door as soon as he's done with you. I mean, the sweet potential husband who's making love to you. Sometimes it's hard to tell the difference between the two, you know.

Here's an easy way to figure out if your emotions are putting a pox on your pole: Masturbate with a dildo inside you. If you get hard then you know you're fucked. I mean, that you've got intimacy issues.

Oh, quick story about dildos. When I was a kid my family was driving behind a garbage truck when a dildo flew out and thumped against the windshield. Embar-rassed, trying to spare my youthful innocence, my mother turns around and says, "Don't worry, honey. That was an insect." I replied, "I'm surprised it could get off the ground with a cock that big."

At any rate, I'd recommend you try four things:

1. **Drugs!** Viagra, Levitra or Cialis, it doesn't matter. Take the smallest dosage your doctor recommends. ED drugs are great at waking up unexplainable penile narcolepsy. Pop the pills in your next couple of ass-hammering sessions, get your dick used to getting hard when you're getting plowed, and then wean yourself off the pills. You won't need them anymore so be sure to mail them to me for safekeeping.

   Don't even *think* about taking these drugs if you have low blood pressure, heart conditions or take medications like nitrates. They'll make your blood pressure fall faster than Britney's career.

2. **Find the Sweet Spot.** It could be that your partners aren't topping you in the way that makes you-know-who spring to attention. The anal canal may be a tube but it's not a straight tube. It's actually S-shaped, with two curves. The angle of entry and your body's position makes a big difference in pleasure. What's the best angle or position? Generally, it's anything that puts your legs at a right angle to your body. Like sitting, squatting, lying on your back or side with your knees pulled toward the chest, or on your knees, "doggie" style. Each of these positions straightens out the S-curve. Experiment with different positions because what works for some people might not work for you.

3. **Pay attention to feelings not thoughts.** You know the saying, "the watched pot never boils?" For you it's "The watched dick never hardens." Meaning, if you're

constantly "standing guard" waiting for something to happen, it'll seem to take forever—if it ever happens at all. Unfortunately, that's when you start ignoring the pleasurable aspects of what you're doing. By keeping your focus on pleasure and forgiving yourself for not getting a raging hard-on, you eventually will.

Question:

As a bottom, I was pretty traumatized by the news that I have hemorrhoids. It was like my ass was telling me it had had enough. The 'rhoids' healed but they sometimes come back. I've bottomed with a few guys since but I'm so worried that my hemorrhoid is going to rear its ugly head that I'm too tense to enjoy it. What do you do when you're a bottom with a hemorrhoid?

– Dying to get laid

Dear Dying:

We'll get you back riding the joystick in no time but first, you need to get yourself to a doctor post-haste-red-hot-QUICK. If you don't you're going to end up needing ass surgery. Like me.

I waited too long to see a doctor after I developed hemorrhoids. Listen to my story and I promise you're going to skip the phone call to the doc and teleport yourself into his office: The doctor points to the "head down, buttocks up" table and asks me to assume the position. When I heard the urethane glove snap on his hands I thought to myself, "Why couldn't I have Attention Deficit Disorder like everyone else?"

My 'rrhoids' were so bad I had to go to a specialist. I almost fainted in his examination room when I saw what looked to be a 2-foot dildo with a gun-like trigger and an open vial of KY jelly. It was a sigmoidoscope. It's inserted into your anus all the way up to your colon. Air is introduced into the scope to aid in viewing. This is the only field of work where pumping air up your ass isn't considered a public relations ploy.

Mercifully, the doctor didn't use the contraption, saving it presumably, for the patients who complained too much about the long wait in the lobby. As I bent over the "bottoms up" table, the doctor spread my cheeks apart as far as he could, giving his lovely blonde assistant an unobstructed view of what I used to think of as a private part. I longed for a shot of dignity the way a diabetic longs for a shot of insulin.

The upshot: Surgery. I had waited too long to get it treated. Three days after the operation, I sneezed. I thought my sphincter had flown out of my ass. The good thing about a hemorrhoidectomy is that you don't really need pain killers after the surgery —the mortification masks most of it.

Just to set the record straight, hemorrhoids are NOT caused by anal sex. In fact, my hetero surgeon laughed at the thought. Seventy five percent of all men will get it at some point in their life. Call me skeptical but I doubt all those straight guys with hemorrhoids are getting ass-hammered at home.

Hemorrhoids are caused by pushing too hard when you're on the toilet. My surgeon doesn't blame anal sex for hemorrhoids; he blames magazines. "The bathroom isn't a library," he said. "Go in, if nothing comes out, get out."

Words to live by.

If you want to avoid my fate—and believe me, you do—then master the secrets of the toilet arts. Never hold your breath when you're on the bowl. It means you're trying too hard. Breathe. Don't effort. Don't strain. Be at one with the bowl. There is no place for struggle in the art of the Zen dump.

Finally, take the magazine rack out of bathroom, drink a gallon of water a day and eat enough fiber to cement the government's food pyramid to the floor.

Question:

I'm an Italian guy living in a big city. I've been involved with a younger guy for a year and our relationship has gone to a level I've never experienced before. I've always been the one to top him, sexually, but now that I've completely fallen in love with him I want to feel him inside me. Unfortunately, my boyfriend is a total bottom. When I fuck him he gets raging hard-ons; when he tries to fuck me he gets raging hard-offs. He can't get it up and he's told me that he's just a bottom and there's no sense in trying to get him to be otherwise.

I'm convinced that this whole top/bottom thing is just a state of mind, a psychological orientation, more than some chronic physical wiring. I think our sex life would be more complete and satisfactory if there was some reciprocity, some versatility in it. Do you think roles in bed can be reversed? How can I make my boyfriend top me? Your kind advice would be appreciated.

– Switch-hitting hopeful

Dear Switch-hitting:

"Kind" advice? You wrote ME for "kind" advice? That's like writing Donald Rumsfeld for "kind" wars. Either way, prepare for a little "Shock & Awe."

Of course it's possible to reverse sexual roles. You just have to ask nicely. My last relationship was getting a little stale so one night I asked my boyfriend if he minded swapping positions for the night. "That's a good idea," he said. "You stand by the ironing board while I sit on the sofa and fart!"

The bastard. And then he wonders why we broke up. Anyway, yes, it's possible to get your boyfriend to "dyke." Meaning, getting a bottom to pass as a top. As in, "did you get him to dyke you?"

Here's how: Talk to him (but never in bed. Bed is the WORST place to talk about sex. Too much pressure. Always talk when you have your clothes on outside the bedroom. That way shame and defensiveness is minimized). Here's what you say: "Honey, I want to get closer to you. I want you to feel what I feel when I make love to you. And I want to feel what you feel when I make to love you. I want to take our love to a higher level."

And then present him with a tiny gift-wrapped box. He'll open it and find a blue sapphire in it. You know, the kind Pfizer makes.

Viagra, the quicker pecker upper, is a wonderful way to take the pressure off him and put his dick inside you. Make sure the box has TWO little blue pills. One for you; one for him. Why? By taking it together, you're re-framing it as an adventure that you'll share rather than a demand that he perform. This way you can share the experience together, make it playful and take the pressure out of it.

The normal dosage for Viagra is 50 mg, but ask your doctor for a prescription of 100 mg pills. It's the same cost per pill but you can cut them in half and save money. Whether it's in your wallet or in your bedroom, always try to get more bang for the buck.

As always, make sure that neither of you has a heart condition or blood pressure issues. Once he gets used to topping you (and liking it) you can wean him off the pills.

You also might want to give Levitra a try. It's Viagra's new competitor. Of course, Viagra's not going to just roll over and, well, you know, take it up the ass. So they're scrambling for a competitive edge. I suggested a brilliant new strategy to their marketing boys: sell Viagra in liquid form and mix it with soda. The new name? "Mount and Do."

No word yet on my royalty checks.

Question:

I'm a 21-year-old college student who gets raging hard-ons for my new crush—
this sweet, gorgeous guy who's exactly what I'm looking for. He wants me to top
him but the second the condom goes on my cock it goes limp. Does this make me
a bottom? I'm getting more and more upset about it, which I'm sure only makes
matters worse. Am I alone in this? Does this happen to others? What can I do to
keep an erection with a condom on?

– **Frustrated as hell**

Dear Frustrated:

You're not alone. I can't think of anything that'll give my dick a flat tire more than
condoms. Well, okay, vaginas, but let's not quibble. Here are the reasons you're losing it and how you can get it back:

1. Focus Interruptus. There you are, kissing, hugging, with his legs around you
ready to be plowed like a snowy Minnesota highway. Your whole body is pounding
with pleasure and anticipation when suddenly you have to switch from passion to lo-
gic. Where are the condoms? Are they in the first or second drawer? And where's the
lube? Do you have enough of it? You stretch to look under the bed and, of course, it's
not there, so now you have to get up to look for it. Ah! There it is! Now look down.
Your dick just went from impressive to impossible. Losing your erection is natural
when your attention goes from the throbbing excitement of sex to the logical pursuit
of safe sex.

Solution: Be prepared. Always keep lube and condoms near the bed. Best bet: Keep a
"fun box" near or under your bed so you ALWAYS know where everything is—and
always within arm's reach. Remember, Preparation = Penetration.

2. Condoms Suck. But HIV sucks even more so we're stuck with the suck. Most of us
have an aversion to condoms because of their awful texture, their medical smell and
that wonderful power they have to reduce sensations.

Solution: Buy buckets of condoms and spend 20 minutes a day for a few days, opening them, stretching them to the breaking point, noticing the different smells and
textures. Do silly things with them like filling them with water, tying their ends and
playing catch with them. Why? To desensitize yourself. To take their power away. By

the time it's 'Showtime' you won't be intimidated by them because the look, texture and smell of the rat bastards will be so familiar.

3. Condoms are awkward. Do you open from top to bottom? Side to side? And then once you've gotten them open, which side do you put on the head of your dick so you can roll it down? Confusion is a great recipe to scare the hard off your on.

Solution: When you're alone, get yourself "excited" and put dozens of different condoms on. Notice they're like socks—there's a right side and a wrong side. How do you know the difference? The "Teat." Make sure you put it on with the teat pointing upward. Also, practice opening them quickly and carefully. *Stellar Tip:* Stick with an easy-to-open brand. For instance, my favorite brand has a slight "V" cut that makes it obvious where to tear it. I notice a lot of condoms don't have instructions or "clues" like a "V" cut, and you can literally try tearing the four corners of the square before you find the right entry point.

The main thing is to become intimately familiar with condoms BEFORE you have sex. That way you'll have power over them rather than the other way around.

Question:

I just read your answer to the guy who loses his erection when he wears a condom. My challenge is a little different. I am negative and always play safe. Love to top and bottom. But when I top, it's really hard for me to cum in a condom. I can go a really long time, but when it's time to cum, I have to pull out and finish it off with my hand. Sometimes it's really hot to shoot my load all over his ass or stomach, but I love to come inside a HOT ass and thrust really deep when I cum. Unfortunately, I rarely get the opportunity. Any suggestions how I can make it happen?

– Trying to Milk it

Dear Milking It:

Most guys who can't "shoot at will" (unless Will is really hot) have a lot going on in their heads. The inability to come in front (or back) of another person is usually caused by shame (like being sexually ridiculed by someone you loved) or trauma (like ending up with the ugly one in a three-way). It's called "ejaculatory incompetence." Can you believe those nut-job psychologists telling us that trauma, shame and ridicule cause this condition and then give it the most humiliating name possible? Grrrr.

Because you can do it some, but not all of the time, I'm going to assume there isn't a

psychological reason for your inability to say the phrase that pays before it sprays ("Oh, God! Oh, God!").

The problem is that your ejaculatory reflex is triggered by the kind of stimulation it gets when you masturbate but not when you're topping. Most of us unconsciously "train" or condition our ejaculatory reflex with very particular types of motion, speed and pressure. Over the years you can "groove" a masturbatory pattern that prevents you from ejaculating inside someone simply because the motion, speed and pressure of fucking doesn't feel the same.

Believe it or not, studies show that men have more intense orgasms through masturbation than fornication. Don't you love that word? It sounds so, I don't know, *Biblical*. Anyway, there's a big difference between masturbating and fucking. And no, it isn't just that there's someone else in the room.

When they're jerking off, most guys instinctively vary the speed and pressure on their penis when they want to cum. But you can't do that when you're topping a guy. Sure, you can thrust harder and faster, but guess what? Most guys don't thrust when they masturbate; they simply move their hands up and down faster.

When you're getting a hand job and you get close to coming, what are you probably going to say? *"Faster! Harder!"* Well, you can't exactly say that to your partner's butt, can you? I mean, you could but I don't really think you'd get much of a response. Most sphincters I know are deaf mutes.

So how do you solve the problem? Simulate the conditions of a good lay when you're masturbating. For example, when you're jacking off, get on your stomach and pretend your hand is your partner's mangina. Cup your hand and thrust your penis into it as if it were a hot piece of "Guy Gap." Yes, you Brits, another reminder to "Mind the Gap."

Keep the position and pressure of your hand steady and use your hips and pelvis to thrust until you orgasm. Like any other type of conditioning, it's not going to work the first couple of times, but keep at it—eventually it will. And once you get it, practice with a condom on. With any luck, your next complaint will be that you're coming inside your partners way too soon.

Question:

Why does everybody think I'm a bottom? The other night I got mistaken for a

bottom by a bottom! How embarrassing is that? I'm talkative, opinionated and loud but people think I'm a bossy bottom instead of a raging top.

Anyway, some magazine compiled a list about what tops should do to be seen as tops. Here they are: 1) Don't talk too much. Good tops should be men of few words. 2) Don't be too energetic. The most rambunctious guys are usually the most effeminate and whoever heard of effeminate tops? 3) Don't pay too much attention to what you wear. You can't be a top and worry about accessories. Wear pants and a shirt that isn't too tight. Steer away from clothing that glitters, anything "big" (buckles, hats, shoes). 4) Don't use the word "cute." 5) Don't wear fruity cologne. 6) Don't shake your groove thang, wiggle your butt to get attention. 7) Be the pursuer, the chaser.

What do you think of the list, Woody? Do you think I should follow their advice?

– Trying to get to the bottom of it

Dear Trying:

Your letter reminds me that gay men are like fine wine: They start out as grapes but you have to stomp the shit out of them until they turn into something acceptable to have dinner with.

Once again, I get a letter asking for advice on how turn a sexual position into a whole identity. And once again, I ask why you feel the need to label yourself. Labels belong on a can not on a man.

Listen to the absurdity of that list. They're saying I can't wear a tight shirt and fuck somebody? I've worn loose shirts, tight shirts, and no shirts and it's never stopped me from doing what I wanted in bed.

And what do you mean, "whoever heard of effeminate tops?" You don't get out much, do you?

Here's my advice: If you're talking to someone you're not sexually interested in and they "assume" you're a bottom (and by "assume" I "assume" you mean he states it), ask him why it's so important for him to know what you like in bed, given that you're never going to sleep with him.

If you're talking to someone you are sexually interested in and he assumes you're a "bottom," why not say nothing and surprise him in bed?

So what if two "tops" end up going home with each other? You say "I'm not into that" and then you figure out what you're both into. Even if it ends up being a mutual hand-job, so what? Wouldn't you rather masturbate someone you're really attracted to than to fuck someone you're halfway hot for?

Question:

I'm 24 years old and pretty experienced when it comes to guys. But I have a prob-lem: Anal sex COMPLETELY disgusts me. Bottoming doesn't appeal to me– I'm not crazy about the feeling, and I can't stay hard when I top because I think it's gross. I was bio/pre-med in college, and am currently in nursing school. I took all those anatomy and microbiology classes; I know what's up there, and it kinda freaks me out. When my partners find out that I'm really not going to top or bot-tom they end up breaking up with me. Why do gay men feel that it's not "sex" un-less it's anal? I'm passionate, romantic, very much into kissing and body contact, but if there's no fucking, I'm kicked to the curb. Should I force myself to do some-thing I hate to keep these guys around? Please help. I'm close to giving up and joining a Tibetan Monastery!!!

– No-Ass For Me

Dear No-Ass:

You're not the only one, man. For years, I refused to top or bottom for the exact reas-on you won't. To me, the male ass was like a vagina—a place where boners go to die. I could no more get it up than I could give it up.

After a few years—okay—a *lot* of years, I realized that my "disgust" wasn't just rooted in legitimate hygiene concerns, but in my uptightness as well. I was like you—wound up tighter than Rosie O'Donnell's girdle. The sooner you realize your discomfort isn't just about hygiene the sooner you'll be able to keep your boyfriends and expand your sexual horizon.

At the most basic level, you have to reframe your perception of the ass as some kind of biohazard. You're a medical student, for God's sakes. If you're squeamish about this I can't imagine what you're going to be like when you're faced with truly disturb-ing events, like gun shot wounds, or worse, me if I wake up next to you.

Here's how to change your disgust into lust:

- **Turn your medical knowledge into practical wisdom.** You have the knowledge of "what's up there" but not the wisdom to wipe it out? Come on! That's like not stuffing a chicken because you know "what's up there." Douches, condoms and Hepatitis shots will wipe out 99% of your concerns. About asses, I mean, not chickens.

- **Demystify your Mystery Meat.** The inability to see your bat cave makes you anal about your anus. It's the great unknown and when something's unknown, you tend to project bad things into it. As opposed to inserting things into it. So, take a shower, clean your back-door winker and grab a mirror. As you look at it from different angles, notice what you're thinking and feeling. Is it gross? Then relax in the face of grossness. It's just a matter of time before you realize, "Oh, it's just a hole."

Next, stroke it with a light touch. It'll stimulate blood flow and make you realize, *"Hey, this kinda feels good!"* Then, gently insert a lubed up finger and follow the instructions in Jack Morin's unfortunately titled book, Anal Pleasure & Health. It's the best book on the subject. The more comfortable you get with the body part that "disgusts" you the more comfortable you'll be about topping or bottoming. Once you handle the hygiene and cork the fear, it'll just be a matter of time before you show—or get—more ass than a Thai whore at a military base.

Question:

I never know which condoms to buy. They all make the same claims. Got any suggestions?

– Snapped to Attention

Dear Snapped:

There are all kinds of hats for all kind of heads. Whatever you choose, keep in mind a couple of things:

1. Squeeze the condom away from the edge of the foil wrap so you don't tear it.

2. Put lube on your dick or on the inside of the condom.

3. Always yell "Incoming!" before entering your partner.

4. Feel the shaft of his cock as it slides in and out of you to make sure it's still on.

5. Get out while you're hard. After you come pull out before you go soft, so the condom doesn't leak semen into him.

6. Don't throw it in the toilet. Condoms can block pipes. Throw it in the garbage or out the door, along with your trick.

Now, as far as the type of condoms, the only way to figure out what's best is to try them on yourself. Here are a few suggestions:

Too Big?

Dream on. But if you really are one of the 6% of men who require a bigger than average condom, then Trojan Magnum XL is your best bet. How do you tell if you need a bigger condom? Slide a toilet-paper tube over your erection. If it slides down to the base of your penis you don't need an extra-large condom. If it doesn't, you need my phone number.

Cum Too Soon?

Try Trojan Extended Pleasure. It's coated with Benzocaine, which dulls the nerves in your dick temporarily. Be sure to put it on correctly. The Benzocaine is on the inside of the condom. Wear it inside out and you'll dull the nerves of your partner's ass. There's nothing worse than getting stuck with a dull ass in bed, so be careful.

Needle-Dick?

Try Contempo Exotica Snugger Fit. It's six percent narrower than regular condoms, making it the narrowest rubber in the market. FYI: condom sizes are based on slurp, not length.

No, wait. My computer keys got stuck. I meant they're based on GIRTH.

Too Dry?

Paradise Super-Sensitive with Astroglide might do the trick you brought home. It's the only condom that comes pre-oiled with a good lube.

Partner Too Frigid?

Try the inSpiral and see if he doesn't spiral out of control. That is, if he doesn't laugh himself off the bed first. InSpiral is shaped like a soft-serve ice-cream cone. Take a lick at it and see what you think.

Fingers Too Wet?

Don't you hate it when you're ready to enter his mangina, only your fingers are too lubed up to open the condom's foil packet? And pretty soon your trick is drumming his finger on your thighs because you're spending more time entering the package than you'll ever spend entering him and by the time you tear it open with your mouth and open the fucker you look down and your hard-on is gone? You know that feeling?

Well, I'll have to take your word for it because that shit's never happened to me.

Anyway, LifeStyles Discs come in sealed plastic containers, like the pats of butter they serve in those tacky diners my ex-boyfriend used to take me to when he was feeling generous and wanted to splurge on me, that cheap fucking bastard, now where was I?

Oh, yeah. Just strip away the top and get to the bottom. It's the very best in "Peel & Bang" condoms.

Room Too Dark?

Try global Protection Night Light, the first government-approved glow-in-the-dark condom. Put the package (the condom, not your dick) near a lamp and the condom will glow for 15 minutes after the lights go out.

Too Selfish?

Try the GOP condom, the Republican Party's first contraceptive. It's made to protect pricks and give the wearer a sense of security when they're fucking somebody over.

Question:

As a former sexual health writer who wrote a bunch of "safe sex" pamphlets and who now works for an organization that promotes condom use I just want to commend you for your honesty throughout the years.

I attended an NIH conference once on condoms. There were rubber experts, human behaviorists, AIDS activists and virologists galore– but after all the talk about rubber's elasticity, it all came down to truths no one was brave enough to utter: Sexual intimacy and condoms are incompatible.

Because like herpes and lung cancer, diseases resulting from human behavior, particularly sexual behavior, are "blame diseases." We can blame somebody for their "risky," "irresponsible," "inconsiderate", and downright unpatriotic behavior. As if sexual desire were a choice. As if it's all about "self control." Anyway, this isn't a question, just a pat on your back for a job well done.

– With you, babe

Dear Babe:

I was with you, GOD, I was with you, until you made that asinine "self control" state-ment.

Of course, it's about "self control." There's never been a disease this awful whose transmission is almost completely dependent on the victim's behavior.

You can't catch HIV from contaminated food like you can with Hepatitis or Polio. You can't catch HIV from another person's cough or sneeze like you can with the flu. You can only catch HIV from consciously performing unsafe sex acts or willfully in-jecting drugs with a contaminated needle. There are exceptions, but the vast majority of infections occur because of personal behavior not impersonal circumstance.

While it *is* about self-control, few people acknowledge the near impossibility of total self-control in something as meaningful as sex. Condoms may be vacu-um-sealed but emotions leak into them. Sex isn't logical, so the decision to wear something that prevents you from experiencing the totality of sex won't be either. We know we should be wearing them but a lot of us still don't, or don't all the time. Not when we're lonely and want a more meaningful communion with another guy, not when drives and feelings and moods meet facts, and figures and stats.

And forget about that "blame" bullshit. When emergency workers pull out dead or injured people out of car accidents, do they "blame" the victim for not wearing a seatbelt that could have saved their lives? If you don't wear a seatbelt and you're seri-ously injured in a car wreck, does that make you unworthy of being helped?

Condoms are like seatbelts—if you don't use them you're taking a big chance of get-ting seriously hurt by an asshole that plows into you. But like car wreck victims, HIV victims shouldn't be accused of malfeasance. It's not a matter of blame; it's a matter of suffering the consequences. And believe me, if you contract HIV because you didn't wear a rubber, "blame" will be the least of your problems.

Just because wearing condoms are difficult doesn't mean "self control" isn't the an-swer. In fact, "self-control" is the only path to staying healthy. The answer is always in the question: "What risk am I willing to take with this particular person in this particular situation at this particular time?"

If you keep asking yourself that question, you'll find yourself using condoms more and more or simply finding more satisfaction in fuckless sex. As a sex advisor it may be impolitic to say that I don't use condoms all the time, but in my mind that makes me worth listening to because I'm not in some Ivory Tower lording it over you hea-thens who can't control yourselves.

I may not use condoms all the time but I use them about 90% of the time and I'm working on the other 10%. Yes, I'm suffering from safe sex fatigue, but you know what? I'm also suffering from plague fatigue and that's a whole lot harder on me than the pressure of putting on a rubber.

Question:

Somebody told me you had a kick-ass column on condoms a while back but I nev-er saw it. Would you repeat it for those of us that missed it?

– A Day Late

Dear Late:

I don't repeat anything except my dinner. Well, okay, some of my partners, too. But I will give you the shortened version:

- Guns offer the best protection against sexually transmitted diseases. Just point it at your partner if he tries to mount you without a condom. If you're scared of guns, try latex condoms. Don't use natural-membrane condoms like lambskin; they're too porous to do a good job of stopping STDs.

- Don't use a condom that's more than five years old. That's about the shelf life of a properly stored condom. Properly stored means they're not exposed to extreme heat, cold or vulgar people who cheat on the people they're cheating on. If the condoms are coated with a spermicide throw them away after three years.

- Never use Vaseline or other oil-based lubricants like petroleum jellies, mineral oils, vegetable oils or cold creams. They'll damage the condoms. Water or silicone-based lubricants are best.

- Don't carry condoms in your pocket. Unless they're the extra large kind. Yes, you'll damage the condoms but at least you'll be showing off and isn't that what it's all about?

- Do not tear the package in half down the middle. That may be fine with ex-boyfriends who screwed you over, but not with condoms. Tear off just the top of the foil.

- Place the condom on the head of the penis and roll it gently down the shaft. Do not pull down tightly against the tip of the penis. Leave a "reservoir," as the experts like to call it, for semen. Don't you love the word "reservoir?" It gives the impression that you're going to cum enough to fill the Hoover Dam when all that'll come out of you is about two teaspoons.

Question:

I am head-over-heels in love with one of my best friends. He is everything I'm looking for in a man. One day we got drunk and he confessed he was in love with me, too. The problem? We're both bottoms and he therefore won't pursue a romantic relationship with me.

Because we are best friends, I know that he's been a top with other men. I used to be a top, but an ex-boyfriend awakened me to the joys of being a bottom, so I've been pretty much exclusively a bottom for the last few years. I recognize that sex is an unbelievably important part of a relationship, but I would hate to miss out on having this wonderful man in my life as more than a friend just because of a preference or silly label. I love my friend so much that I would do anything to make him happy, but I'm having trouble awakening my inner top. Any advice?

– Topless in Atlanta

Dear Topless:

You label queens kill me. You'd give up your soul mate because he's not the right bed bait? Call me weird, but I'd rather jerk off with someone I love than fuck someone I don't.

Here's a novel idea—why don't you date first and figure out the sex later? You guys don't have a prayer of getting together unless you stop confusing sexual positions with personal identities. I mean, read your letter again. It's full of "I AM a bottom" and "he IS a bottom" rather than "I prefer bottoming" or "he likes to get penetrated."

See, it's easier to expand a behavioral preference than to change a psychological identity. So the first thing you've got to do is reframe what you consider an identity into what it really is—a sex act. Then and only then do you have a shot at making the changes you want.

Here's what I recommend:

Prioritize. Sex may be important but it's not what keeps couples together. Ask any-one in a long-term relationship. You guys didn't just make sex the most important criteria for having a relationship, you've made it the *only* one. How about knocking sex down a peg or two on your hierarchy of importance? You're so concerned with sexual compatibility that you haven't given any thought to dating compatibility. Just because you're good friends doesn't mean you'd make good lovers. Get some ro-mantic experiences under your belt before you reach for his pants.

Diversify. You're both acting as if fucking is the only acceptable thing you can do in bed. Ever heard of blowjobs, hand jobs, rimming, finger-play, shall I go on? There's a lot more to sex than sticking it in a hole and banging away. Although don't mention that to my fuck buddies. I don't want them getting ideas.

Believe in Change. You said yourself that you enjoyed topping and then switched to bottoming. Well, you changed once. You don't think it can happen again? Here's my two-word reply: Puh-leeze.

Lovers often go through phases where one is completely into bottoming or topping. Then they reverse, or shift from one to the other, depending on the mood or situ-ation.

Different people in different situations bring out different sexual appetites. Neither of you might want to top each other *today,* but you're a fool if you think your feelings won't change as the relationship changes. If love can move mountains what do you think it can do to bedrooms?

Medicate. If you want a jump-start, try Viagra or its competitors a couple of times. Just make sure you don't have a heart or blood pressure condition. Sometimes all it takes to hit a homerun is a chance at bat.

Question:

My boyfriend and I are both healthy, monogamous and HIV negative. He wants to stop using condoms but I'm not sure that's such a good idea. He's insulted be-cause he thinks it's a sign I don't trust him. I don't know what I think but my gut says no. Am I wrong?

– Worried About Safety

Dear Worried:

Okay, picture this: You're a Siamese twin. Your lover, attached at your shoulder, is a bottom. You're a top. He's going to cheat on you tonight. You only have one ass.

My point, and I do have one, is that only Siamese Twins know if the person they're attached to is going to cheat. In fact, studies show 25% of married men have cheated on their wives at some point. Gay men? I don't even want to go there. I don't mean to be pessimistic because there are lots of monogamous couples, but people are human. They make mistakes. They have a sincere intention to keep their word but they often don't. They change, you change, circumstances change. That's why you have to ask yourself this fundamental question if you want to resolve your dilemma:

Knowing there's a high probability that one of us is going to cheat at some point in the relationship, am I willing to take the risk?

Now, before you answer consider these factors.

1. **What's your partner's sexual history?** Did he have an odometer on his bed when you first met him or was he "reasonably promiscuous?" For the record, I subscribe to the male ego definition of the word—*You're promiscuous if you've had sex with more partners than I have.* Seriously, history is the best indication of the future. If he was an indiscriminate meat-starved nympho before he met you, chances are greater that he's going to cheat than if he was "reasonably pro-miscuous."

2. **What was your partner's view about condoms when you met him?** When you first asked him about a condom did he say, "No, I live in a house"? Or did he know what they were and insisted on using them? If he didn't, and he ends up cheating, he's likely to do it without a condom, putting you at great risk.

3. **How easy is it for you and your partner to talk about sex?** The more difficulty you have talking about it the more likely one of you is going to do the No Pants Dance with a stranger. Communication is the best way to trick-proof your marriage. If you go deaf, dumb and blind on the subject it's just a matter of time before one of you walks in on the other and says, "Honey, that better be me you're fucking or we're through!"

4. **How sure are you that he's never going to cheat?** Read Malcom Gladwell's *Blink*. Unless you're a paranoid drama queen, don't listen to "reason" or facts when you're gut tells you something different. Point your intuition meter at his crotch. Does it point to safety or bust a coil?

5. **If he does cheat, how sure are you that he'll use a condom?** Maybe you can live with him wandering from time to time, but will he wander safely?

Even though I was monogamous in my last relationship (don't ask me how *that* happened; it shocked the hell out of me, too) we both agreed to use condoms. We saw it as buying a life insurance policy. We bought it not because we were *certain* that something was going to happen; but in case it did.

But that was us. Every couple needs to decide for themselves.

Question:

I'm a 20 year-old voracious bottom. I've tried all kinds of lubes and none are equal to my industrial-strength fucking. What do you think is the best brand for us eager bottoms?

– Dried-out bottom

Dear Dried:

Before we get into this, can somebody please tell me why lubes are called "personal"? Is there a "public" lubricant I don't know about?

Picking a lube is like picking a good trick—You want something that goes down easy, isn't smelly or hard to get off you.

I've tried what some experts call "the best lubes" and hated them, so there's no point in telling you which lube I like best. You're better off test-driving the different brands and seeing for yourself. Here's what to look for:

Texture & Smoothness:

You don't want your *personal* lubricant to be sticky or tacky. You want your lube to be as slippery as your boyfriend when he's confronted with the strange underwear you found in the back of his truck.

Dryness:

Did the lube disappear after the first few strokes —like the commitment-phobe you dated last year? Or did it stick around like that trick last night that couldn't take a hint?

Container:

May sound stupid to use this as a criteria but if it takes two hands to squeeze out a few drops it ain't worth it. You want the thing to be so easy you can open it with your feet. I'd stay away from jars and tubs—they tend to collect pubic hair—a double-yuck factor in my book. Try some of the new "Anal Shooters" developed at the National Gay Chili Cook-off. Actually, they're suppositories that come in 5 ml applicators. Talk about a lube with staying power!

Wash-off Factor:

If you're looking for convenience, forget about oil-based lubes like Vaseline, baby oil or Crisco. They not only destroy condoms, but they're so hard to get off you'll have to pressure-wash your ass. Trust me, you're not that big of a bottom.

Taste & Smell:

Believe me it's important. Do you really want to screw with a lube that smells like ass in a butcher shop?

How long it lasts:

You don't want a "premature ejaculating" lube. Meaning, three strokes and it's over. You want a long-lasting lube so you don't have to keep re-applying it.

Irritation Factor:

The two ingredients that cause most skin irritations are Nonoxynol-9 (which you should NEVER use because it promotes HIV infection) and glycerin (a form of sugar that makes lubes taste sweet). Well, three if you count tricks who keep calling you by the wrong name. So, if you've got sensitive skin use lubes made out of botanical in- gredients. Or change your name.

Temperature:

Some of the newer lubes create heat or cold when you rub it on. You know, like the guys you take home—they can give you heat stroke or freezer burns.

Main Ingredient:

There are basically three kinds of lubes: Water-based, oil-based and silicone-based. Each has their pluses and minuses. Silicone lasts longer but it's a lot more expensive and you need soap and water to get it off. Plus, you CANNOT use them with silic- one-based toys. You'll cause a chemical reaction that'll ruin your prized butt-plug.

Water-based lubes may not last as long but you hardly need any soap with the water to wipe off. And unlike silicone lubes, they're not going to grow your butt-plug a third eye.

Bottom line? If you want a lube with a great fudge-packing quotient, then test, test, test.

Don't spend a fortune doing it either. Buy sample packs that have a wide variety of brands.

Question:

How's it going? I read your column all the time and I get such a kick out of your responses. I want you to know that I always defend you. I always tell my friends "He's not a heartless bitch, he's a cranky bastard. There's a difference." Anyway, I have a question. Can you explain the safe/proper way to use butt plugs (other than sticking it up your butt?). Do you use it just before sex or are you supposed to leave it in you for a few hours? If so, is that safe and does your butt become loosey goosey afterwards?

– Anal Retentive

Dear Anal:

You call me a bastard and then ask for mercy? Christ, you sound like my dad right before I shot him.

And what was that crap about "other than sticking it up your butt?" Where else would you stick a butt plug—in your ears?

Butt plugs are toys so there aren't any "rules." What feels right for you may not feel right for someone else. There's two reasons to use them: Because they stimulate the anal opening (science for "it feels good!") or as a sort of training device to get your sphincter muscles ready to take on larger cargo.

Remember, the sphincter has two muscle rings. The first is voluntary (you can squeeze them at will—it's what stops you from taking a dump when you read this column). The second is involuntary (you can't consciously control it—it's why you can't stop from taking a dump when you read this column).

It's that second ring, the involuntary muscle (less than a quarter inch from the outer voluntary one) that causes most of the pain in anal sex. If you can relax it you're in for a great ride. If you can't, you'll punch your partner into the next room.

The idea of anal sex is to scream for more not yell for help, so "training" the inner sphincter muscle to relax is critical. That's where butt plugs come in. If you keep them in long enough, the inner sphincter muscle relaxes on its own (muscles can't stay contracted forever—at some point they have to release).

You're going to have to use more than a butt plug to stretch the inner muscle if you want painless anal sex. So gradually introduce bigger and bigger dildos until you can insert one the size of your partner's penis without pain.

Let me say that again, WITHOUT PAIN. Remember, pain is a signal that something's wrong. You know that burning sensation you feel when you're taking in your partner? It means you're stretching the sphincter too much and causing micro-tears. God help you if you're not using a condom because you just created a transmission route and put yourself at major risk for HIV. If you do it right (lots of elasticity training of the sphincter) you shouldn't have any pain during anal sex. Discomfort maybe, but not pain.

Question:

I hooked up with a horny, passionate guy a few times recently and want to ensure that I give him the best screwing possible. Luckily, I have great staying power when I'm topping him (sometimes too long, but that's a "problem" for another time). Got any advice on how to drive bottoms wild? I want to keep this guy around!

– Considerate Top

Dear Considerate:

We'll get into tactics in a minute but first a warning: Good techniques make good technicians. It's passion that drives people crazy. Why do you think Latin lovers have the reputation of being great in bed? Because they're skilled workers? No, because they're passionate and that passion leads them to trying new things and doing them well.

Now having said that, there *are* ways to make your sessions so hot his ass will set off the smoke detector. It basically comes down to how you thrust. This is the most im-portant of all techniques and the least understood, due in large part because of what I call "Jackhammer Porn." Since most of us watch porn and it almost always shows machine-like fucking, we sort of "learn" what they teach: Vary the positions but not the pace.

Thrusting patterns are important because the law of diminishing returns says pleasure is inversely related to repetition. You know how the first few bites of a great steak always taste better than the last few? It's because you didn't pause, take a sip of wine, or a bite of a side dish. Taste buds get sensitized easily. So, do manginas. Mix things up a little so that that the taste buds in his rectum don't get sensitized. Okay, did that last sentence make anybody else nauseous? Because I'm about to blow chunks.

Anyway, here are some classic Tantric sex techniques that'll keep those rectal taste buds on high alert:

The *"Thrusts Of The Heron"*: If it were a law, I'd call it, Three Thrusts And You're Out. You go in deeply for three consecutive thrusts, and then go in very shallow.

The *"Thrusts Of The Dragon"*: This is basically tripling the Three Thrusts and You're Out Rule. You thrust deeply nine times and then once shallowly. You can also do the reverse: Thrust shallowly for nine times, then once very deeply.

The *"Thrusts Of The Phoenix"*: Okay, this one takes some math, so skip it if you got confused by the book, "Subtraction: Addition's Tricky Friend." Basically, the pattern is 9 deep/1 shallow, 8 deep/2 shallow, 7 deep/3 shallow, and so on until you reverse it and get to 1deep/9 shallow.

Other thrust patterns: Alternate slow and deep with slow and shallow. Or try the "Mouse" technique: Quick and shallow thrusts. Then of course, there's The Eagle: hold your penis motionless at the entrance of his starfish then swoop in quickly and deeply. But for heaven's sake, do this AFTER you've been screwing for a while. Otherwise, it'll hurt so much your partner will knock you into the fall elections. Which will hopefully stay Democratic because I don't know who can take all that Teabagger ass-hammering. Talk about jackhammer thrusts! These people must be awful in bed —the same exact thrusting pattern night after night for seven years. Is anybody else's ass sore?

Again, these are general rules—different thrusts for different butts, I always say. The whole idea is to vary the stimulation. Do that and his butt hole will blink "Welcome!" in Morse Code every time he sees you.

Question:

I'm an 18-year-old freshman in college. I met the guy I'm in love with at the gym

pool where I spied the perfect amount of hair disappearing into his Speedos. Everything between us is great except... we're both tops!! Early on he said, "We have a predicament..." I told him the solution was clear– we fuck EACH OTHER. That night, after repeated refusals to wrap his legs around me, which resulted in a sweaty wrestling match, I said, "This is your predicament, not mine. What about reciprocity?" He claims that he enjoys bottoming 'in theory' but 'in practice' he has never enjoyed it. HOWEVER, his dick throbs like mad whenever I finger him and I knoooow he enjoys it. But whenever I actually go to make a move, he clamps up and stops me.

I let him penetrate me a few nights ago, in a hope to speed up the reciprocity... and still no luck. I'm scared that his refusal is a sign that he doesn't really love me. I don't let anyone penetrate me– I only do it because I love him. I'm not accustomed to this fear of losing somebody (I usually get the impression that people like me too much, not too little, as cocky as that may sound). I'm wondering, could it also be the age thing? He's 24...I was wondering if in your infinite wisdom you had any advice for how I should handle the situation?

– Bottomed out

Dear Bottomed Out:

No, it's not about age. Christ, I have underwear older than your age gap. And no, his refusal to bottom isn't a sign he doesn't love you. It's a sign you have the seduction skills of a clock-watching butcher. Read your letter again. Does it sound like you're seducing him or raping him?

You can't pressure somebody who has issues about bottoming without making them more defensive and resistant. And believe me, your boyfriend has more issues than People Magazine's archives.

Leaving aside hygiene concerns and real preferences, a lot of guys subconsciously think they'll lose their masculinity if they bottom. They're afraid it'll make them "the girl" in the relationship. That they'll end up loving it so much that's all they'll wind up wanting. They're afraid they'll be emasculated, tagged as a "bottom," and be the butt of humiliating jokes.

So your boyfriend is filled with fear, worry and anxiety and what do you do? Harrass, pressure and nearly assault him. Oh. My. God.

Here's what you need to do:

1. **Call a time out.** No bottoming, no topping, no talking about either. Tell him you've approached it the wrong way and you want to take the issue off the table for a while to concentrate on the things you both like to do. Let the pressure you've built up dissipate.

2. **Be vulnerable.** Reintroduce the subject by telling him the fears *you* have about bottoming. Trust me, you have them. Whether it's a perceived loss of masculinity or what I call the Martha Stewart syndrome*—we all have issues about it. Do NOT use this as a short cut to his short hairs. This is about talking and listening. Leave the action for later.

3. **Use my proven Get Him to Roll Over® system.** It's a 5-step plan to replace the cement in his heels with helium. It's in my column titled, "How To Get Your Boyfriend To Bottom." Send me an email and I'll send you the column.

Question:

I've been with this guy for a few months now, and things are moving along quite nicely with one exception. We're both tops. We click on so many levels except that one. To avoid a stalemate in the bedroom, I've been bottoming every time, but I really want to switch things up. I've asked him but he won't. Is there any way I can change his mind?

-Wanting to top

Dear Wanting:

Yes, with my proven <u>Get Him to Roll Over System</u>*. Here's how it works:

1. **Seduce; Don't Confront.** You can't argue your way into a man's starfish. Try it and the ten-foot fence around his sphincter will grow to twenty. Confront him and he'll electrify the fence. Instead, seduce him. Even a salesman knows you don't go for the 'close' right away.

2. **Drop the labels.** Saying something like, *"I'm not going to be the bottom in this relationship"* will trigger every emotional hot button he's got about his masculinity. Instead, tell him you're crazy-attracted to him and want to experience different aspects of him. Make it about Desire and you'll fill his heels with helium. Make it about who's the woman in the relationship and you'll fill them with cement.

3. **Emphasize Compromise.** Remind him that partners don't just do things *to* each other in bed, they do things *for* each other.

4. **Get a Commitment to Considering It.** You'll never get a highly resistant guy to say, "I'll do it." But you can easily get him to say, "I'll consider it." Here's how: By promising that as you move slowly to the Main Event (see next point) you will not try to top him under any conditions. This will get rid of his "anticipatory anxiety"—constantly being on guard that you're going to trick or force him to bottom as soon as he lets down his guard. Trust is a key issue—don't violate it, or you'll spend the rest of your sex life on your back memorizing ceiling patterns.

5. **Use Your Sexual Power.** You have power over him. It's called Desire. Use it. What turns him on about you? Your chest? Walk around the house shirtless more. Does he like the way you grunt in bed? Grunt more. The more you turn him on the easier it'll be to turn him over.

6. **Desensitize his Ass.** Start by simply laying on top of him stomach to stomach. Do NOT lift his legs as if you're about to enter him. Kiss and touch all you want but be on top. Once he gets comfortable with that, then advance progressively:

   ◆ *Ask if you can rim him.* Rimming is nothing but the back door of a blowjob —and feels about as heavenly.

   ◆ *Gently brush the head of your penis against his sphincter.* Don't use your hands; otherwise he'll think you're going to pull the old "I'll just stick the head in" trick.

   ◆ *Slowly push between his legs so that the length of your dick presses against his perineum.* The heat and hardness of your dick against such a sensitive area will flood him with pleasure. The idea is to get him used to having your dick touching his Demilitarized Zone without freaking out.

   ◆ *Slowly rub the shaft of your penis against his perineum in gentle thrusting motions.* Basically, it's stimulation by simulation.

After a few weeks, when you sense he's receptive ASK him if you can make love. The combination of his love and desire for you mixed with the respectful and sexy way you've gone about it will almost always result in a "Yes."

Question:

In a recent column you wrote, "Tops get HIV all the time." When you use "Top"

in that sentence, are you referring to a person who identifies himself as a top or are you referring to the act of penetrating the anus of a sexual partner? The reason for my question is that I am unaware of any reported cases of a man contracting HIV from penetrating a vagina. Similarly, I was not aware of any reported cases of a man who never engaged in anally receptive sex contracting HIV from penetrating the anus of another man. Are you aware of numerous cases of men contracting HIV solely from penetrating the anus of other men?

– **Looking to make decisions with all the right information.**

Dear Looking:

You've never heard of a man contracting HIV from penetrating a vagina? I've got one word for you: Africa. And one number: 25 million (infected). And one percentage: 43% (the portion of AIDS made up by "tops" or men).

Now what was your question again?

Oh, yeah, that tops don't get HIV. Well, men don't like to have morals get in the way of having their way, so why should facts? But if you're in a listening mood, here's what you need to hear: The second most common way of getting HIV is to be the top in rubberless sex.

True, the risk isn't anywhere near being the bottom in condomless sex, but it's still pretty risky. Some respected scientists put the chances of catching HIV at 1 in 50 if you're bottoming and 1 in 500 if you're topping (without a condom). But the truth is no one really knows. And trust me, you don't want to be the guinea pig who finds out.

So here's why tops are at risk if they don't put the jacket on:

1. During the excitement of sex, what with all the endorphins and adrenalin rushing around, you're less likely to feel micro-abrasions or scrapes on your dick.

2. There is almost always blood inside a man's hole, even in bottoms who've fucked so much they have an odometer in their sphincter. That's because tearing almost always happens during sex. And don't forget, 75% of all men, gay or straight, will have hemorrhoids. Don't be fooled by the fact you can't see the blood— sometimes they're invisible specks that never leave the anal canal.

3. Whatever's inside a butt (blood, fecal matter) is going to go inside your "piss slit" and into your urethra, which is lined with soft mucous membranes that tear easily.

4. Do the math: 1+2+3=HIV

Question:

I certainly appreciate what you said about fucking and pain and cocaine a few columns back, butt for me it's pot and the better the pot the bigger the dick I like up my ass. And this is from a top... Without the "lubrication" from marijuana I become one of those bottoms who after 5-10 minutes says, "Stop, it hurts!" (Not the kind of bottom I like to fuck.) Not that it really hurts but I just don't like it all that much sober. Any comment on sex stoned?

– High

Dear High:

How many times do I have to tell you people that masking pain with drugs is asking for trouble?

You know that burning sensation you get when you're penetrated by someone bigger than you're used to? It's a signal that you're ripping the lining of your anus. You don't feel it when you're on drugs or alcohol because they distort or dull the senses. You may be causing unnoticeable but very real internal bleeding. And God help you if you're getting fucked without a rubber in that kind of circumstance. You might as well phone your doctor and ask him when you should start the meds.

I never "recommend" that people use or not use drugs. What I recommend is that if you choose to use them, use them wisely. Using them to get a bigger dick up your ass is not using them wisely. It is, as I'm fond of saying, falling off the stupid tree and hitting every branch on the way down.

As far as why you only like getting fucked when you're on drugs, I'd take a hard look at the labels you used and the sneering way you used them. It's obvious that you have some deep-seated issues about getting penetrated. The marijuana puts you in just enough of a fog to drop your defenses.

Usually, it's a fear of losing your masculinity by doing something associated with women—getting penetrated by a penis. It's a form of passivity that scares macho guys to the core. Let's face it, the worst thing you can call a guy isn't "fag." It's "girl."

How do you get over it? The same way you get over anything—you do it till it doesn't bother you anymore. It's called desensitization. For you, that means putting yourself in uncomfortable but not panic-provoking situations—like bottoming without drugs. Eventually, you'll master the anxieties you have about losing your masculinity.

There's a famous film that sex therapists-in-training watch to understand the power of desensitization. A guy who's extremely uncomfortable with saying dirty words is given a sheet of paper filled with the kind of words my editor yells whenever he sees me. He (the guy in the film, not my editor) starts off blushing and stammering. For 20 minutes, he keeps saying the words and at the end of the film, you can see that he's become completely comfortable. "Dirty words" had no power over him any-more. They were just syllables strung together in a certain way.

So, my advice to you is, desensitize yourself. Force yourself to bottom without drugs. In fact, make like a pizza—get pounded into dough and tossed up high. A LOT. To the point where the meaning you've associated with bottoming disappears. You're like the guy in the film—only you're uncomfortable with bottoming, not dirty words. Once you understand that you don't lose your manhood when you bottom, your need for drugs will disappear.

Question:

Sometimes I feel like I'm weird because all my friends prefer fucking to oral sex. I would so much rather give head than fuck or get head than get fucked. Do you think I'm weird?

– The mouth that roared

Dear Mouth:

One of the reasons many men, straight or gay, prefer oral sex is that we're visual creatures. Whether you're fucking an ass or a va...va...vagi– Christ, I'm so gay I can't even say the word.

Anyway, you can see more dick with blowjobs. With anal sex you can't see shit.

Well, actually...

Alright, bad metaphors aside, with blowjobs you can see all of your dick (or his) go in and out. You can also see more of your partner's body.

Even if there wasn't an "explanation" for your preferences, why feel weird about them? There's very little choice in sex. You don't get to choose which gender you like; you don't get to choose which member of the gender you like; and you don't get to choose what you like to do with the member of that gender. I say quit trying to justify your preferences and get busy doing them.

Question:

Settle a bet. When it comes to oral sex who is the top and who is the bottom? I'm a top when it comes to anal but I love sucking dick; so, am I an oral bottom? Or am I a versatile top? Is "top" and "bottom" only in reference to anal? If active is the top and passive is the bottom then the guy doing the sucking should be the top but a lot of guys I've chatted with don't see it that way. Who's right?

– Confused

Dear Confused:

I rarely describe people as tops or bottoms unless I need to make a point quickly. Labels belong on a can, not a man. They encourage people to make whole identities out of sexual positions. So if you label yourself a "bottom" it isn't just that you like being penetrated—it brings up a whole set of stereotyped personality characteristics that have negative associations.

Think about it—when was the last time you heard a joke about a "Top?" But you hear plenty of derogatory comments about "bottoms." Like, "there's nothing but bottoms in this town." Or, "I'm not going to be the bottom in this relationship." I mean, when was the last time you heard somebody say, "Oh, him? He's nothing but a big top." So, basically you're asking somebody who hates labels to promote them.

HOWEVER.

I'm intrigued by your question. And after doing a lot of thinking, here's where I come down on it (pun intended):

If you're doing the sucking, you're being the bottom.

Here's why: "Top" and "bottom" are modern labels for masculine and feminine. Ancient Greeks and Romans celebrated homosexuality AS LONG AS YOU WERE THE TOP. Or rather, as long as you didn't do what women did in bed.

And what did women do in bed? Receive a penis—in their mouth or between their legs. Therefore, any "Man" who received a penis through oral or anal penetration was considered feminine, woman-like, and put himself in danger of being ridiculed, ostracized and in some cases, physical harm.

A woman does not have a penis, so she has to do something to it or for it. That leaves giving head and getting fucked. So, if as a man, you're giving head or getting fucked, you're taking the role reserved for women. Or if you insist on labels, being a bottom.

Another example: Hyper-macho men who can't accept their homosexuality rationalize their man-on-man action by saying, "Hey, as long as I'm the one fucking I'm not gay," or "As long as I'm not giving head, I'm still hetero." In other words, as long as I don't do anything to or for a penis, I'm a man.

So, yes, if you're into labels, you would be an anal top and an oral bottom. But that takes us back to my original premise: Who cares about labels? You can go down on a guy and depending on the situation, feel dominant (male) or submissive (female). Same with bottoming. You can be a submissive bottom or a dominant one. My God, have you ever been with "power bottoms?" You are SO not in charge. You're just the human dildo along for the ride.

So, stop worrying about labels. When it comes to oral sex, the only thing I'd worry about is teeth.

Question:

I'm an ass-freak. I love to 'toss salad' and get my own lettuce flipped and licked. I want my sphincter in porn-quality shape– the pinkest pink possible. Have you heard of 'anal bleaching?' I want to get it done, but where? It's not the kind of thing salons advertise. Also, is it possible to DIY it?

– Throbbing for love

Dear Throbbing:

You're shit out of luck. There are only two salons I know of that do it—one in Australia and one in Los Angeles called Pink Cheeks, which has a sign hanging on the wall that says, "NO WHINING." Funny, I have the same sign hanging over my bed.

Here's how the backdoor beauty regimen works: You clear the area of any hair, then apply bleaching creams with the active ingredients used in photo processing and rubber manufacturing. Ahh, smearing toxic chemicals on my ass—now there's a procedure I don't get nearly enough of. Anyway, you then use the cream each night until you achieve the desired lightness. Professional butt-bleachers claim you'll see results in one to two weeks.

I'm strongly opposed to anal bleaching. First, who's going to know? How many people are going to look at your starfish with enough light to tell the difference? Are you expecting guys to say, "You know, there's something different about you but I can't put my finger on it?"

Second, and more importantly, medical experts believe the active ingredients in anal bleach creams are toxic. Basically, you'll be rubbing flammable chemicals on your butt. I'm all for having 5-alarm sex but do you really want flames shooting out of your ass like a rocket on take-off?

If you're going to pursue a perfect shade of ass no matter what I say, then at least look for creams that don't have Hydroquinone or Mercury. There's only one bleaching cream with non-toxic, natural ingredients. And no, I'm not going to tell you what it is because I don't want your ass on my hands.

Wait. That didn't come out right.

Anyway, shaving your ass may not get your sphincter in porn-quality shape, but it's a whole lot safer. A bald starfish heightens sensations and improves sanitation (the sur-rounding hair catches hot-from-the-oven bum-bons. Shave the hair, save the wall). You have two options to make that happen:

• Depilatory Creams

Use only the ones marked "for sensitive areas." Remember, products like Nair are c-h-e-m-i-c-a-l-s. If there's no hair left to dissolve because you've left it on too long it'll start dissolving your skin. So, if it says "leave on for two or three minutes" you better stare at the stopwatch as if the ticker's going to detonate your dick.

• Shaving

Do NOT use an electric shaver—you'll mulch your sphincter. I shouldn't have to say it, but I've learned to never under-estimate gay stupidity: Do not wax the hair off your ass. Your screams will shatter all the windows in the house. For best results, follow the instructions in my column about shaving your balls. Here's the short version: Cut the extra long hair with scissors, take a warm bath to open the pores, spread your legs wide, and shave. *Carefully.* You don't want the tub to look like you botched an abortion.

Question:

I'm a famous bottom from way back and my doctor said I should consider getting an anal pap smear because I'm a candidate for anal cancer. Is he kidding me? Can bottoming cause cancer?

– Sitting on pins and needles

Dear Sitting:

Here's the test to see if you should get an anal pap smear: You're in bed. It ain't Thanksgiving. Your tricks keep saying, "Whew, that's one terrific spread!"

In other words, RUN, don't walk and get smeared. Research shows that men who engage in receptive anal sex are 30 times likelier to get anal cancer than those who don't. And if you're HIV-positive you're at an even higher risk.

Anal cancer, like watching a Fox reality show, can burrow so far into your ass you won't know if you're breathing or farting. It's also fatal (the cancer, I mean. No word on the Fox programming). The cancer can be caused by the human papillomavirus (HPV). Most sexually active gay men carry this virus, which tends to lie dormant and causes no harm. As many as 90% of HIV-positive gay men carry the virus.

If you keep hearing, "Do you think you'll be able to handle all these people at once?" and it's not your father talking to your mother about a dinner party, you need to get an anal pap smear every two or three years. That's if you're HIV-negative. If you're HIV-positive, you need it annually.

Question:

My boyfriend has incredible stamina and he often remains hard after he's orgasmed. Because he often cums before I do I want him to stay inside me when he's fucking me until I can cum myself. But he's afraid that ejaculations can cause a condom to break so he pulls out. Now I don't know about the rest of your readers, Woody, but when I'm bottoming and I want to cum, I want my partner's dick inside me, not laying on top of me. Can he stay inside me and still be safe?

– My Turn!

Dear My Turn:

Actually, the condom is less likely to break after he cums in it. Here's why: It lubric-ates the latex, protecting it from tears.

There's another reason, too. Most erections decrease in size and firmness after ejacu-lation, further decreasing pressure on the condom.

Still, he's right for pulling out. With more lubrication on the inside and decreased girth from orgasming the condom won't fit as well and it's more likely to slip off. And oh, dear, there goes his milk all over your cookies.

You have two options: 1) Teach him how to last long enough for you to blow some wattage (there are standard techniques for delaying ejaculation. Look it up in the web or look at some of my past columns). 2) "Double-bag" him. Have him wear two rubbers. It'll decrease his sensation so he can last longer and keep you safe at the same time. But Dear Lord, who wants to wear two rubbers? I vote for option #1.

Question:

I enjoy anal stimulation during masturbation and sex, and have noticed my rectum often produces a clear fluid when I insert a finger or toy in it. When I have an orgasm, the fluid becomes more copious, almost as if I had ejaculated back there. It even looks and smells like semen. What's the mystery liquid?

– Smell my finger

Dear Smell:

Your ass—unlike a vagina—is not self-lubricating. There's moisture in the anus but there are no glands capable of producing fluids when you're getting plowed or doing the job yourself.

The stains on your sheets are probably a combination of several different bodily flu-ids. First and foremost, sweat. When things get hot you perspire. Sex gets us excited and all worked up. Unless you're a republican. Then *someone else's* sex life is what gets you all worked up.

Depending on what position you're taking on the matter, sweat could run together and collect near your anus.

Second, the motion of anal stimulation (in and out and in and out—you know, like most men trying to decide whether they want to be in or out of a relationship) draws fluid from the rectum to the opening of the anus.

Third, yer lube. Personal lubricants heat up from the combination of friction and body heat, which makes them runnier, foamier, and sometimes creamier than normal.

Again, will somebody please tell me why lubricants are "personal?" I mean, the last time I asked for a "public" lubricant the guy behind the counter just scratched his head.

But then again, I shouldn't be asking these kinds of questions at a fast food joint. Especially when the guy behind the counter is my father.

Question:

In a recent article you said that bareback topping is the #2 avenue for HIV infection, with bareback bottoming being #1.

That statement concerns me. My physician is a prominent gay doctor and I am a personal friend with another physician. Both have told me the same thing: The chances of a barebacking (BB) top (strictly top, not one that bottoms occasionally) being infected with HIV from barebacking is equal to the risk of unprotected oral sex – taking cum in the mouth and swallowing. My physician goes so far to say that bottoming with a condom is no riskier than being a bareback top! With the exceptions that condoms can leak and break and assuming the top doesn't have open sores on his penis.

Now both doctors qualify this by saying they don't want to give the impression that a BB top is 'safe', but they also concede that the gay community has a misconception that oral sex is 'safe', when the fact is there are documented cases of HIV transmission thru oral sex, a fact the gay community still wants to deny. Thus they don't encourage BB topping or unprotected oral sex where the guy getting sucked could be poz. But I think the gay community needs to be properly informed. While the risk of BB topping is extremely low, in reality it's no riskier than unprotected oral sex.

– **Straightening you out**

Dear Straightening:

You need a new doctor and better friends. Any doctor who says that the risk of top-ping without a condom is equal to giving oral sex needs their license to say "beauti-cian," not "Doctor of Medicine."

As long as there are no scrapes, cuts or abrasions in your mouth the risk of giving oral sex, even if a positive guy shoots in your mouth, is minimal to non-existent. However, the risk of topping somebody who's positive is much greater, even if you don't have any sores or cuts on your penis. Here's why: As you thrust the opening of the urethra (the "hole" in your penis) is stretched open, allowing fecal matter, blood particles and other delicious goodies to enter the urethra. As you pull out for the next thrusts, the urethral opening closes, pushing all those goodies deeper into the ur-ethra, possibly scratching or tearing the urethra and creating a transmission route.

Contrast that to giving head. Somebody (hopefully hot) thrusts himself into your mouth. If there's no scratches or abrasions in either his penis or your mouth how can the virus enter your bloodstream? There is the possibility that it could be absorbed through the soft lining of the mouth's membranes but there's also the possibility that I'll go on a date without putting out. The odds are about the same: next to nothing.

Let me tell you a parable that speaks to your doctor's prominent stupidity:

Before the Iraq war started, Saddam Hussein sent George Bush a letter. Bush opened the letter and it contained a message that was obviously in code:

370HSSV-0773H

George W. couldn't figure out the code so he sent it to the CIA. They couldn't solve it so it went to the NSA and the FBI, then to MIT and NASA and finally to the Secret Service. Eventually, they asked an elderly WWII code breaker. The guy took one look at it and said, "Tell the President he is looking at the message upside down."

That's a long way of saying your doctor is looking at HIV research upside down. Hand it to him right side up and get a new doctor.

Question:

A lot of new guys I pick up haven't cleaned or douched before I top them. I have a pretty nice looking member and sometimes a bottom gets too eager and leaves his calling card on me. Now, I go soft at the sight of brown lining a guy's hole or on my condom-wearing penis. Sometimes I suggest we play in the shower, or ask if

he needs to take a shower. But sometimes the date's answer is that he's "fine" when he isn't. Asking a bottom to shower isn't as simple as it may seem— and particularly inappropriate if he's the one who's hosting. What's a tactful way to ask somebody if they've douched?

– **No Surprises**

Dear No Surprises:

What kind of skanks are you bringing home? Most guys know the potential embarrassment of leaving tire tracks so they'll clean up or decline to be entered.

Your guys don't seem to give a crap.

Of course, it could be inexperience, not apathy. Most *experienced* guys have the good sense to say, "Not tonight, dear, I'm a ticking shit bomb." Or something like that. But inexperienced guys, especially if they weren't planning on bottoming that night, might not say anything. They might suspect they're not "fresh" but still play the odds with you. Or they may think that rubbing a little extra soap in the area earlier that night will keep the muds at bay. Either way, inexperienced guys are the least likely to voice their concern, especially if they don't want to miss out on a sausage-sitting opportunity.

And here's the thing—experienced or not, douched or not—accidents happen, so don't freak out. After all, it's just crap, the by-product of digested food. Don't act like it's some bio-hazard that's going to grow you a third eye.

The solution? Ask, don't hint. In a playful but emphatic way. Rub yourself on the outside of your date's bat cave and say, *"Are you prepared for this kind of sex or should we do something else and wait for another time?"* If you wanted to be more direct (and judging by the blockheads you bring home, you do), you could say, *"Is your backside clean enough to have sex or do you want to wait for another time?"*

If they say they're as clean as a nun's conscience and you get a squirt of hamburger helper anyway, stay calm. Say, "Don't worry, it happens to everybody at some point. The best way to prevent it is to douche with plain water."

Final Thoughts.

If you follow the instructions in this book you will be able to inhale living room furniture through your anus like it were a line of coke. Or a porn star. This might make you want to bottom for the entire western world but I'd like to offer a cautionary tale against doing it with inappropriate people. Meet my friend, Doctor Dave. He could never bottom until he read this book. He wanted to try his newfound skill on multiple partners but he worked 14-hour days at his practice, so he didn't have the opportunity to meet a lot of people. Unfortunately, he ended up having sex with several of his patients. He tried to rationalize his behavior by reminding me that he was single, that his patients were single, that he wasn't the first doctor to sleep with his patients and that nobody was harmed by the experiences. Finally, he asked for my advice.

I said, "Dave, *you're a vet.*"

My point, and I do have one, is a) never take your pets to Dr. Dave, and b) don't take sex so seriously. Let this story remind you that no matter how serious sex gets, there's always room for laughter. Thank you for allowing me to help you experience a better sex life. Now, go. Bottom like a porn star. And don't forget to laugh.

ABOUT THE AUTHOR

I started my career as an op-ed columnist for *Southern Voice*, a gay newspaper in Atlanta. Upset that I won the city's Most Loved Columnist three times in a row, I rallied when I also won the Most Hated category. The editor then approached me about writing an irreverent sex advice column. I thought, "Awesome! Send me your cutest employees and I'll get started!" We syndicated the column all over the country and I sort of became known as the "East Coast Dan Savage." I then went on to write my first gay sex book, *Men Are Pigs But We Love Bacon* (Kensington).

My proudest achievement came a few years ago when I helped create a website that helps parents come to terms with their children's sexual orientation. We get thousands of emails a year from parents and their gay children thanking us for making it possible for them to reunite as a family. If you or someone you love is going through drama and strife about being gay, please visit us at www.familyacceptance.com.

Oh, wait, back to my bio! Soon I was writing gay themed pieces for *Newsweek*, *The New York Times*, salon.com and other publications. I also became a frequent commentator for National Public Radio's All Things Considered. That led to a major production company in London asking me if I'd like to audition for a co-hosting role in a heterosexual sex makeover series called *The Sex Inspectors* (they thought it'd be cool to put the gay in it). With the screen test cameras rolling, I remember the production chief asking me what I thought of women faking their orgasms. "That's nothing," I sniffed. "Men fake whole relationships."

I got the job.

The show went on to be an international hit, airing in 12 countries, including the U.S. on HBO. It led to my biggest book yet, *Sex Inspectors Master Class: How To Have An Amazing Sex Life* (Penguin).

Once during filming, I sat on the bed with a woman I was advising (don't worry, we were fully clothed—it wasn't that kind of show!). The video cameras that we put throughout her house showed how cruelly she rejected her husband's advances. I said, "Put your arm around me, I want to show you how you reject your husband." I whacked her arm away like it was an unwanted fly and looked away from her. Indignantly, she said, "I do NOT do that!" I said, "Yes, you do." She knew I was right. I could see her face softening. I leaned in. "Can I tell you a secret?" She nodded. I cupped my hand around her ear and whispered something. She started bawling. The producer, director and audio people went nuts because the microphone didn't pick up what I said. The director stopped the filming to give the woman time to compose, took me aside and asked, "What the hell did you say to make her cry like that?

I said, "*Men have feelings, too.*"

I love giving advice to people. I love to see barriers crack and humanity come to the surface. I hope I was able to do that with the book you're holding in your hands and that you've enjoyed reading it as much as I did writing it. Shoot me a quick email and let me know if you have any questions or comments: Mike@woodpeckermedia.net. Or visit me at http://www.gaydatingsuccess.net.

All the best to you!

Printed in Great Britain
by Amazon